此丛书系国家中医药管理局国际合作司"中国中医药国(境)外传播系列资料编译"项目。(项目编码 1603050400004)

The Series belong to the project of State Administration of Traditional Chinese Medicine of P. R. China. (Proj. No. 1603050400004)

U0138272

GENERAL TCM KNOWLEDGE OF SURGERY & OSTEOLOGY & TRAUMATOLOGY

LI NAIQING

CAO JIANCHUN

CHINA PRESS OF TRADITIONAL CHINESE MEDICINE

• BEIJING •

General TCM Knowledge of Surgery & Osteology & Traumatology
Professor LI Naiqing
Department of Surgery, Dongzhimen Hospital Affiliated to Beijing University of
Chinese Medicine
No. 5 Haiyuncang, Dong Cheng District, Beijing, China
100700

©**China Press of Traditional Chinese Medicine, Beijing, China, 2005**
No. 28 East Road, Beisanhuan, Chao Yang District, Beijing, China(100013)
President Tel: (86-10)64405720
Press Tel:(86-10)64065415/84042153,Fax:(86-10)64405719
Home Page:http://www. cptcm. com, E-mail: cptcm@cptcm. com
Published by China Press of Traditional Chinese Medicine.
Distributed by Beijing Issuing House, New China Book Store.
*
Format:787×960 1/16　Printed Quantities:10　Word Count:114000
First Edition:December 2005　First Printed:December 2005
Price:RMB Yuan 20. 00
*

V

General Foreword

Traditional Chinese Medicine (short as TCM) is the splendid traditional culture of the Chinese nation, which has made outstanding contributions to the prosperity of the Chinese nation. Moreover, it has developed a school of its own in the field of traditional medicine and pharmacology of the world. TCM plays an important role in health undertakings not only in China but also in the world.

TCM is a science studying the law and regulation of human body's living activities and alteration. It embodies profound recognition of life science of human body, which is scientific and progressive. The health concept and clinical practice reflect the trend of modern science.

TCM includes a set of complete and unique theoretical system. With practical effects, it accumulates abundant experience in diagnosis and treatment of all kinds of diseases. As the excellent representation of traditional medicine in the world, TCM takes unique superiority in the diagnosis and cure of various diseases, especially for some modern difficult and complicated cases, such as cardiovascular disease, diabetes, tumor, immune disease, viral infective disease, and it is playing a much more important role.

In the 21th century, with the transformation of medical mode, the pedigree of diseases alters. Iatrogenic and aging diseases are gradually increasing. People's consciousness of prevention and health is promoted and the need for raw medicines in the international community is increasing. As a result, there will be more room for the development of TCM, contributing greatly to human's health.

In order to promote TCM culture forward in the world, State Administration of Traditional Chinese Medicine of People's Republic of China (SATCM) carries out the project. The compilation and translation of this set of popular science series is also part of it, in which we will introduce the basic knowledge of TCM. This series includes 12 books, covering the Brief History of TCM, Basic Theories of TCM, Chinese Tuina, Chinese Herbs and Formulae, and so on. And it has vivid language and colorful illustrations, which helps the readers at home and abroad comprehend correctly the basic knowledge of TCM in a short time, familiarize the application of TCM in health and disease prevention, so as to fit modern people's pursuit for high qualified health life.

State Administration of Traditional Chinese Medicine of

P. R. China

December, 2005

Preface

As we all know, surgery of western medicine (WM) takes operation and manipulation as the main method in the treatment of trauma, inflammation, tumour, malformation and other diseases. Then what diseases do the surgery, osteology and traumatology of traditional Chinese medicine (TCM) study on?

Surgery of TCM study suppurative infection on body surface, breast, goiter, benign tumour, cancer, dermatosis, anus, rectum, male external genitalia, and peripheral vascular diseases, trauma, abscess of internal organs(such as carbuncle of liver, acute appendicitis), acute abdomen, hernia, and urinary system and sexual transmitted disease. The osteology and traumatology of traditional Chinese medicine investigate on trauma and osteopathy.

If you want to know something about surgery of western medicine, let's review its development.

The surgery, osteology and traumatology of TCM have a long history. Descriptions on bones or tortoise shells in Shang Dynasty recorded some of surgical disease names.

Surgery became an independent special course of study in Zhou Dynasty (1066A. B. ～249A. D). Huangdi Neijing recorded the etiology and pathogenesis of the superficial infection and pyocutaneous disease, and proposed toe amputation in the treatment of finger or toe gangrene. Hua Tuo of late Han Dynasty use Mafusan as general anesthetic in the operation of bone sequestrum excision. Gong Qingxuan's liu Juan zi Guiyi Fang(483A. D.) of Nanbei Dynasty is the first surgery monograph. It recorded the management of trauma at that time. In Sui Dynasty, Zhubing Yuanhou Lun (610 A. D.), written by Chao Yuanfang, described the suture of broken intestine, the repair of abdominal hernia, using silk in the ligation of vascular. Qianjin Yaofang (652A. D.) of Tang dynasty, written by Sun Simiao, recorded the manipulative reduction of mandibular dislocation, which was similar to that in modern medicine, and application of urethral catheterization that employed fistular onion leaf to resolve urine retention and was 1200 years earlier than that of rubber tube in French at 1860. In Jin and Yuan Dynasty, Shiyi Dexiao Fang (1337 A. D.), written by Wei Yilin, recorded aconite root, Dature and so on were used as anaesthetics before bonesetting; and suspension repositioning in the treatment of spine fracture. In Ming dynasty, Waike Zhengzong, written by Chen Shigong, described that silk—thread should be used to sew the incision of windpipe cut off by the suicide. Special department of treating bone fracture and disarticulatus was set up in Qing dynasty.

The plentiful treating experience of ancient times has been developed and boosted greatly. Now please let me introduce it to you briefly.

This subject has gotten great advancement since the establishment of the People's Republic of China. In clinical aspect, some research findings achieved by the department for special course of study or special diseases have reached the world level. Since the beginning of 1950s, the prevention and treatment of acute abdomen by combination of TCM with western medicine has been developed widespread and achieved some therapeutic results.

The treatment of chronic osteomyelitis by Chinese medicine and combined treatment of traditional Chinese medicine and western medicine gained significant result, especially to the formed bone sequestrum, bone cavity empyema, formed sinus tract, it has unique therapeutic efficacy.

In the aspect of breast diseases, the treatment of plasma cell mastitis, areola mammae syrinx, and cyclomastopathy has obtained great advancement.

By combining external treatment and endoscopic therapy,

operation and intervention with needle, the peripheral vascular disease has been treated with good curative effects. It has high curative rate not only for earlier period of disease but also for later period of disease, and has very low relapse rate and mutilation rate.

The research of burnt chiefly personified at the respect of scab — enhancing and moist — exposing therapy, which was different from Western medicine.

The treatment of hemorrhoids and fistula diseases developed greatly. Application of discission — ligation therapy solved the difficulty of treating high position anal fistula. Extra — stripping and intra — ligation was a refining operation of combined hemorrhoids. Injection of Xiaozhiling sclerosing agent in the treatment of internal hemorrhoid proved effectively.

TCM methods of treating internal hemorrhoid and chronic prostatitis were effective. Clinical and experimental studies on male infertility and sexual disturbance have gained great achievement.

The treatment of malignant tumour can lengthen life span, improve living quality and adjust immune function of the body. The combination of Chinese medicine with operation, radiotherapy, and chemotherapy can promote postoperative recovery, reduce the side effect of chemotherapy, and improve therapeutic efficacy.

Based on the experiences in osteology and traumatology of TCM and modern scientific knowledge and methods, the workers in osteology and traumatology have summarized eight new manipulations of bone — setting, and developed new external splintage. They have developed a set of new therapies for fracture in which oral medication of Chinese herbs, and external treatment and functional exercises are taken in combination. They set forth therapeutic principles of treating fracture, i. e. , combination of movement and rest, paying attention to both bone and tendon, both external and internal treatment and cooperation of doctor and patient, gaining a good result of quick healing of fracture, good recovery of function, less suffering and complications. This made treatment of fracture go up to a new level.

In the field of dermatology, many gratifying results have been gained; and TCM methods have improved the curative effect of dermatomycosis, eczema, and dermatitis. For connective tissue diseases such as systemic lupus erythematosus, Tripterygium wilfordii preparation can lessen symptoms and adjust immune function.

In recent years, in order to ameliorate AIDS patient's symptoms, improve living quality, prolong live span, pharmacologists have tried to screen drugs from Chinese herbs.

LI Naiqing

Contents

Chapter1 Surgery of TCM

1. 1 Pyocutaneous Diseases ·· 1

  1. 1. 1 Local Infection ·· 1

  1. 1. 2 General Infection ·· 11

1. 2 Mammary Diseases ·· 14

  1. 2. 1 Mammary Infectious Disease ···························· 14

  1. 2. 2 Breast Mass ··· 17

  1. 2. 3 Mammary Tumour ··· 18

1. 3 Wart ·· 21

  1. 3. 1 Meat Wart (or Exophthalmic Goiter) ·············· 22

  1. 3. 2 Lapis Wart (Thyroid Carcinoma) ···················· 23

1. 4 Tumour (liuyan) ·· 24

  1. 4. 1 Blood Tumour ·· 25

  1. 4. 2 Cocoon Lips ·· 26

  1. 4. 3 Cervical Carcinoma ······································· 27

  1. 4. 4 Kidney Carcinoma ··· 29

1. 5 Anorectal Diseases ·· 31

  1. 5. 1 Hemorrhoid ··· 31

  1. 5. 2 Anal Abscesses ··· 34

  1. 5. 3 Anal Fistula ·· 35

  1. 5. 4 Anal Fissure ·· 36

1. 6 Urinary And Male Diseases ···································· 38

  1. 6. 1 Male Sterility ·· 39

  1. 6. 2 Chronic Prostatitis ·· 40

  1. 6. 3 Prostatic Hyperplasia ····································· 42

1. 7　Peripheral Vascular Disease ·························· 44

　1. 7. 1　Shank Sore ································· 44

　1. 7. 2　Gangrene ································· 46

1. 8　Other Surgical Diseases ························· 48

1. 9　Dermatosis And Sexual Transmitted Disease ·············· 51

　1. 9. 1　Tinea ···································· 51

　1. 9. 2　Damp Sores ····························· 53

　1. 9. 3　Psoriasis ······························· 56

　1. 9. 4　White Crust ····························· 58

　1. 9. 5　Red Butterfly—like Sore ·················· 60

　1. 9. 6　Syphilis ································· 62

　1. 9. 7　AIDS ·································· 64

Chapter2　Osteology And Traumatology

2. 1　Fracture ································· 68

2. 2　Dislocation ································· 73

2. 3　Soft Tissue Injury ··························· 75

2. 4　Injured Internal Syndrome ······················ 77

2. 5　Bone Disease ································· 79

Chapter 1 Surgery of TCM

1.1
Pyocutaneous Diseases

The pyocutaneous diseases are purulence diseases caused by various kinds of etiological factors, which are similar to infectious diseases in modern surgery. They can be divided into general infection and local infection. Local infection can be divided into furuncle, carbuncle, pyogenic infection of muscle, hard furuncle, erysipelas, acute lymphangitis, deep-rooted carbuncle, gravity abscess, crewels, tuberculosis of bones and joints, etc. General infection can be divided into carbuncle complicated by sepsis and inward sinking.

Let us see the clinical manifestation and treatment of them.

1.1.1
Local Infection

1.1.1.1
Furuncle, Carbuncle, pyogenic infection of muscle, tipped carbuncle
【Diagnosis】

Furuncle, carbuncle, pyogenic infection of muscle and tipped carbuncle are all acute suppurative diseases in the superficial position of the muscle and skin, characterized by a local reddened tumefaction with burning sensation and pain in most cases. Furuncle is the same disease in both TCM and WM; Carbuncle corresponds to superficial abscess and suppurative lymphadenitis of WM, characterized by shinning tumefaction, sized 6~9cm. Pyogenic infection of muscle developed from soft part of the body suddenly, manifested by reddened tumefaction spread wildly, burning sensation and pain, accompanied by obviously general symptom. Tipped carbuncle generated form tenacious and thick part of the skin, sized over 9cm. These diseases can be divided into three stages: formation, suppuration, and exfoliation according to pathogenetic condition. Formation stage manifested by red swelling, burning pain and functional disturbance; Suppuration stage we can see signs as local abnormal protrusion swelling, intensified pain, pain as a chicken pecking, keep our hands on lump, we can feel it soft on the central and fluctuation, that is pus being formed; Exfoliation stage, the lump rupture and discharge purulent fluid. Disease of excess type discharge tenacious and yellowish purulent fluid while deficient type discharge tenuity purulent fluid without new granulation tissue grown in the sore.

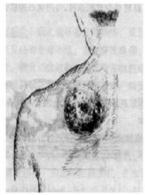
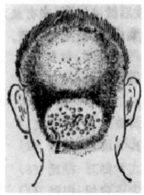

Figure 1 Carbuncle on The Back

Figure 2 Tipped Carbuncle on The Neck

【Treatment】

Internal treatment: ①In the formation stage, expelling wind and clearing heat, removing toxic materials and dampness method are used. For high fever and hydrodipsia, add Gypsum Fibrosum (sheng shi gao), radix trichosanthis (tian hua fen). For convulsion and syncope-syndrome add Angong Niuhuang Wan and Zixue Dan. ②In he suppuration stage, if the suppurating prolong, promoting pus drainage method and the preparation Tounong San can be used. ③In exfoliation stage, if the pus disperses too much, the proper method is replenishing qi and blood, Sijunzi Tang for deficiency of qi and Bazhen tang for deficiency of both qi and blood.

External treatment: ①In the formation stage, clearing heat and subsiding swelling method is followed, Jinhuang San, Yulu San are used for external application, or Qianchui Gao, Taiyi Gao mixed with Hongling Dan or Yangdu Neicixao San to cover the lump. ②In the suppuration stage, it is advisable to discharge pus by an incision. ③Exfoliation stage, at the beginning, pus drainage and removal necrotic tissue method should be followed, Ba'er Dan or Jiuyi Dan and drainage with medicated strip are used; after all pus is out, Shengji San mixed in the sore, covered with Taiyi Gao and Shengji Baiyu Gao.

On the whole, suppurative disease in the superficial position of body, with a local reddened tumefaction with burning sensation and pain, can be treated in accordance with these dis eases.

1. 1. 1. 2

Facial Hard Furuncle

Facial hard furuncle is an acute suppurative sore on the face. It is similar to the scope of facial furuncle and carbuncle in WM. Characterized by millet-grain likes sore, with hard and deep base, feels like nail. The head is the confluence of all Yang meridians, if virulent fire is concentrated, it is easy to induce carbuncle complicated by sepsis and threatens life.

【Diagnosis】

Initial stage: it is manifested by millet-grain pus at the beginning on the face, itching or numb, gradually develop to red swelling and burning pain, sized 3~6cm, with deep and hard base, just like a nail, aversion to cold with fever to heavy patient.

Middle stage: 5~7 days after morbidity, we can see swelling spread gradually, infiltrating to circumference obviously, aggravating pain, pus point breaking, accompanied by fever, thirsty, dry stool, brown urine, reddened tongue, yellowish and greasy coating, slippery and rapid pulse.

Later stage: 7~10 days after morbidity, it can be seen swelling being limited. The top elevated, the base turn to soft, purulent fluid discharged, pus embolus outflow with the pus, swelling getting extinct, pain stopping, general fever failing. Patients get recovery 10~14 days later, it is favorable case. But facial furunculosis, especially on ala nasi, upper labial part, easy develop to general infection (Zouhuang), manifested by depressed cacumen, dark colour without pus in the ulcer, with dark red colour in surrounding skin, swelling extending without limited, even led to head, face and five sense organs swelling seriously, accompanied by high fever, restlessness, coma and delirium. The mal-management includes absurd crushing, careless bruising and too early sectioning.

【Treatment】

(1) Internal treatment Clearing heat and dispelling fire, cooling blood to remove pathogenic heat. Wuwei Xiaodu Yin, Huanglian Jiedu Tang, Xijiao Dihuang Tang with modification is used in the treatment.

(2) External treatment In the initial stage, encircling toxicant and reducing swelling. Jinhuang San, Yulu San or Qianchui Gao are applied, or Liushen Wan, Zijin Ding bruising and blend with vinegar; When pus is formed, it is effective using pus drainage and removal of necrotic tissue method. It is advisable to mix it with Jiuyi Dan or Baer Dan on the top, and then cover the lump with Yulu Gao and Qianchui Gao. If the pus exudes un-smoothly, we drain with medicated strip. Fluctuation can be felt in the cen ter, it is necessary to incise the furuncle and discharge purulent material. After diabrosis, pus drainage and removal of necrotic tissue, promoting tissue regeneration and wound healing method should be applied. Jiuyi Dan and external cover with Jinhuang Gao are mixed in the ulcer. If the pus is over, Shengji San can be used and Taiyi Gao or Hongyou Gao can be applied to the surface.

1. 1. 1. 3

Erysipelas / acute lymphangitis

Erysipelas is an acute infection with the skin flare up suddenly, the colour just as overlain cinnabar. TCM and WM call it erysipelas both. Acute lymphangitis happens on the four limbs. Red thread like lesion on the skin can be seen, and it spreads upward quickly.

【Diagnosis】

Erysipelas usually occurs on the leg and face. At the beginning, it is manifested as aversion to cold with fever, headache, bone aching, then little red spot is seen on the skin and flares up to large area with clear boundary, slightly higher than skin surface. If you press it, the red will fade; raise your hand, it will turn red again. There are peliosis, petch, ecchymosis, blister, and blood blister on red swelling of the skin of serious patient, even cutaneous diapyesis necrosis.

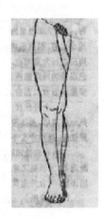

Figure 3   Acute Lymp angitis on The Lower Limb

Acute lymphangitis often takes place on the inner part of four limbs, usually with case history of extremity hard furuncle or skin damaged. There is local reddened tumefaction with burning sensation and pain in extremity hard furuncle first, then red thread like lesion can be seen on inner part of forearm and leg, extending to the trunk and stopped in the elbow or axil on upper limbs, and in the popliteal fossa or groin on lower limbs. There are aching lymphadenectasis in axillary fossa, popliteal fossa pars inguinalis.

【Treatment】

Internal treatment: Cooling the blood, clearing heat-toxin and Puji Xiaodu Yin is used for acute lymphangitis developed on the head; Longdan Xiegan Tang for happened on the chest, abdomen, waist and groin; Wushen Tang add Bixie Shenshi Tang for disease on the lower limbs; Xijiao Dihuang Tang for erysipelas of infant with toxicant inward sinking.

External treatment: Jinhuang San or Yulu San are used for external application; Seven-star needle or three-edged needle are applied in swift pricking blood therapy; blood letting and detoxifying, cover the wound with Taiyi Gao mixed with Hongling Dan.

1.1.1.4

Deep Carbuncle

Deep carbuncle is a general designation of acute purulence diseases of bone and joint. This chapter introduces suppurative osteomyelitis and osteomyelitis with perforation around Huantiao(GB30) point, which is similar to purulence coxarthria.

【Diagnosis】

There is severe acroaesthesia in the initial stage of suppurative osteomyelitis, then gentle red and heat on the skin, bone swelling, deep tenderness percussion pain on extremities; The pus is formed 3～4 weeks later; In exfoliation stage, the pus is thick at first, then turn thin, dipping wet continuously. The ulcer is difficult to heal. Sinus will be formed. The bone sequestrum can be touched.

Osteomyelitis with perforation around Huantiao point manifested as pain at bones and muscles near the hip, limitation
of activity; aching and swelling aggravate close behind, fluctuation can be felt in some patients with high fever; pus is
discharged after exfoliation. Because of the bone is damaged, healing is not easy. It will cause joints abnormal,
stiff, or joint dislocate and get disabled.

Tc—MDP, ^{67}Ga bone imaging can help doctors giving early
diagnosis. X-ray, CT, nyxis will assist the giving of diagnosis.

【Treatment】

Internal treatment: in the initial stage, clearing heat and dissipating dampness, removing blood stasis and obstruction in
collaterals, Huanglian Jiedu Tang add Wushen Tang are
used; In the purulence time, clearing heat and dissipating
dampness, harmonizing ying and expelling toxicant, we can
use Huanglian Jiedu Tang add Xianfang Huoming Yin; After rupture of the ulceration, regulating and replenishing qi
and blood, clearing and dissolving remnant toxicant, Bazhen
Tang add Liuwei Dihuang Wan should be applied.

External treatment: In the initial stage, it is advisable to use
Jinhuang Gao or Yulu Gao for external application, use
splint or plaster stone to fix the affected limb or joint; In the
purulence stage, it is advisable to discharge pus by an incision; After rupture of the ulceration, it is advisable to apply
Ba'er Dan or Qisan Dan medicated strip in drainage, and

cover it with Hongyou Gao or Chonghe Gao. Bone sequestrum should be removed. If there is sinus formed, it is advisable to use Qianjin San or Wuwu Dan medicate paper
string to enlarge the opening of sore, then drainage with
medicated strip, or apply debridement.

1.1.1.5
Crewels and Tuberculosis of Bones and Joints
The scrofula is a chronic purulence disease developed around
the cervical part. Tuberculosis of bones and joints is developed in bones and joints, the liquor puris can flow to tissue
space near the lesion, and form abscess. Once the abscess
ruptured, the pus is like phlegm.

【Diagnosis】

Scrofula: At the initial stage, lymph node of neck gets
swelling, which is tenacious, boundary obscure, increasing
gradually, adhere to skin, or attach to each other. At the
later stage, after cutting open or breaking itself, we can see
pus mixed with catkins like matter, the opening of sore like
hidden cavity with murky grey granulation tissue on the
sore, blue colour around the sore, or there is sinus
formed.

Tuberculosis of bones and joints: The patient often has tuberculosis case history in other part of the body, especially
tuberculosis. It is mostly seen on vertebrae, then hip-joint,
knee-joint and ankle-joint of lower extremity, then shoulder-
joint, clbow-joint and wrist joint of upper extremity. Initial
ly, it is manifested as joint pain, functional impairment. In
the middle stage, the joint gets swelling obviously, surrounding muscular atrophy, abscess formed near or far away

form the lesion. After rupture of the abscess, the pus flows out with catkins like matter, and long time after the rupture, the opening of the ulceration will get depressed, with blue colour around the sore, or form sinus which is difficult to cure.

Tubercle bacilli could be found in the cultivation of pus. Tissue biopsy is helpful to the final diagnosis.

【Treatment】

Internal treatment: Using Kaiyu San for syndrome of Qi stagnation and phlegm coagulation, Liuwei Dihuang Wan add Qinggu San for syndrome of hyperactivity of fire due to yin deficiency, Xiangbei Yangrong Tang for syndrome of deficiency of both qi and blood.

External treatment: In the initial stage, it is advisable to cover the tumour with Chonghe Gao or Yanghe Jiening Gao mixed with Heituixiao, change it every 5~7days. In the intermediate stage, cover the lesion with Chonghe Gao. If the pus is not formed, it should be changed to Qianchui Gao. If the pus is formed, it is advised to cut open to let out pus and necrosis tissue. At the later stage, it is advisable to use Wuwu Dan in pus drainage and removal necrotic tissue. If the pus is exhausted, Shengji San should be used to promote the cure of the ulcer. If there is hidden cavity or sinus, it is advisable to use Qianjin San to enlarge the ulcer or apply ligation therapy.

1. 1. 2
General Infection

1. 1. 2. 1
Carbuncle Complicated by Sepsis

Carbuncle complicated by sepsis and inward sinking developed in the Yang Syndrome of ulcer and sore, for over flaring of toxic heat or deficiency of resistance energy, which lead to dangerous syndrome of toxicant pathogen disperse, invading the Zang-Fu. It is similar to general acute suppurate disease of WM. The disease succeeding hard furuncle is called carbuncle complicated by sepsis, otherwise called inward sinking.

【Diagnosis】

Carbuncle complicated by sepsis often with a hard furuncle case history, it is manifested as sinking and turning dark on the sore tip without pus formed in the primary lesion suddenly, the lump being tenacious, spread quickly, with obscure boundary, missing protecting boundary, the colour of skin turning dark red. The general syndromes are chilling, high fever, headache, restlessness, chest distress, or accompanied with nausea, vomiting, diarrhea, or coughing, breathlessness, bloody phlegm; or with ecchymosis, urticaria, jaundice, et. al, even appearing coma.

【Treatment】

Internal treatment: Wuwei Xiaodu Yin, Huanglian Jiedu Tang, Xijiao Dihuang Tang three preparation are combined and modified, adding Zixue Dan or Angong Niuhuang Wan for comatose patient; adding fritillariae tuber, snakegourd root for patient with hemoptysis; adding fresh bamboo juice for patient with cough and dyspnea; adding raw rhubarb (decocted at later stage), mirabilitum dehydratum (administered after dissolved); adding gambir plant, dens draconis, Indian bread with hostwood for spasm and faint; adding raw rhubarb (decocted at later stage), raw cape jasmine fruit, artemisiae capillaries for jaundice.

External treatment: To the place of sinking and turning dark on the sore tip, it is used with Baer Dan, and coving Jinhuang Gao, spreading on Jinhuang San or Yulu San concocting with cold water to ferrule and moistening it without intermission. Others may be referred to the external treatment of primarily hard furuncle.

Other treatment: it may be utilized with large dose broad-spectrum antibiotic in the initial stage; maintaining fluid and electrolyte balance; giving disposal aiming directly at symptom; Qingkai Ling 40ml, intravenously guttae after being diluted, once daily.

1. 1. 2. 2
Inward sinking

Inward sinking is an danger and urgent disease developed in the Yang Syndrome of ulcer and sore, because of healthy energy deficient interior, over flaring of toxic heat, which lead to toxicant pathogen disperse, vital Qi cannot conquer pathogen, toxicant can't disperse outside but invade inside, settled in nutrient and blood, transfer into Zang-Fu. Patient with tipped carbuncle easy to suffer the disease, so it is called deep-rooted carbuncle toxicant invagination. It can be divided into three kinds according to the stages of the disease: fire inward sinking, non-festering carbuncle, and asthenia ulceration.

【Diagnosis】

It is more often to see it in elders, or diabetic patients. The local sign is the tip of the sore being not too high or depressed, swelling evenness, dispersed, the colour of the ulcer is dark violet and gloomy, there is little pus or no pus. Purulence is thin and sometimes with green colour. Carrion is cast off but the surface of the sore turns white and shining, with no granulation grown, with scorching aching sense or indolent.

Constitutional symptom: high fever, chilling, or without fever, headache, restlessness, or depressed, even coma and delirium, dyspnea with rapid respiration, or with faint breath, chest distress and pain, cough and bloody phlegm, nausea and vomiting, abdominal distention and pain, constipation or diarrhea, excessive sweating and cold limbs, or syncope with convulsion, jaundice and so on.

All in all, fire inward sinking is the extreme of heat pathogen; Non-festering carbuncle is the syndrome of asthenia of healthy energy and over abounds of pathogenic factor; asthenia ulceration is caused by Yang deficiency of spleen and kidney or Yin deficiency and frustrated of stomach.

【Treatment】

It is advised to use integrated traditional and western medicine

Internal treatment: For exuberance of pathogenic factors and intense heat syndrome, Qingying Tang add Huanglian Jiedu Tang, Angong Niuhuang Wan or Zixue Dan with modified should be used; For deficiency of vital Qi and exuberance of pathogenic factors syndrome, it is effective to use Tuoli Xi-aodu San, Angong Niuhuang Wan; For yang deficiency of both spleen and kidney, it is advisable to take Fuzi Lizhong Tang; For yin deficiency and frustrated of stomach syndrome, Yiwei Tang is the most common decoction.

External treatment: refer to that of tipped carbuncle, other therapy to carbuncle complicated by septicemia.

1.2
Mammary Diseases

Many kinds of diseases occur in the breast, and all of them are called Mammary Diseases. It happens in the male and female, but female is more than male.

1.2.1
Mammary Infectious Disease

It includes specific infection and non-specific infection. The former can be divided into breast carbuncle and phlegmonous mastitis etc. The latter can be divided into mammary tuberculosis etc. The various infections are cured unsuitably can develop as mammary fibroadenoma.

Breast Carbuncle

It refers to an acute suppurative disease caused by invasion of heat-toxin into the breasts.

【Diagnosis】

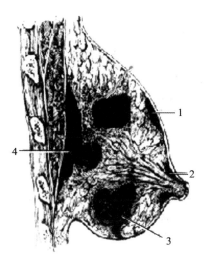

Figure 4　Breast Carbuncle
1. Superficial Abscess
2. Subareolar Abscess
3. Deep Abscess
4. Abscess Mammary

This disease often happens in the ladies during lactation. In the initial stage, there is swelling and pain in the local breasts, no red (slightly red colour) in the skin, no heat (slightly heat) sensation in the skin, or companied obvious general symptoms, such as aversion to cold and fever, nausea, vomiting, slippery and rapid pulse. Formed pus(middle stage), palpable enlarged mass in the breast ,obvious tenderness, or pain in the local area with red colour and burning pain in the skin, and palpable enlarged lymph nodes on the same side, even softened mass with fluctuant sensation when touched by fingers, punctured absorption has pus, accompanied by severe symptoms. After rupture, cheesy pus after rupture of breast carbuncle, with heat relieved after pus discharge, then progressively healing of the wound.

In the routine Blood examination: The total count of peripheral leukocyte and neutrophil ratio are obviously enhanced. B type supersonic wave findings can help to diagnose the deep abscess.

【Treatment】

Internal treatment: Qi accumulated heat syndrome, accompanied distending pain in the breast, swelling and pain in the breast. Formulae, modified Gualou Niubang Tang ; Heat toxin hyper-activity syndrome, swelling and burning pain in the breast, burning sensation in the skin of the mass with obvious tenderness, Formulae, modified Tounong San, Body deficiency and Toxin lingering Syndrome, thin pus after rupture, relieved tumefaction and pain but difficult to be healed and easy formed the mammary Fibroadenoma, Formulae, modified Tuoli Xiaodu San.

External treatment: In the initial stage, it is advisable to apply heat compress and Tuina the breasts to promote the discharge of stagnant milk. Using Jinhuang San or Yulu Gao or Liusheng San plus Vaselin externally on the infected area, also can put sterilized cloth into 50% Mirabilite liquid and apply it on the breast. After pus is formed, it is necessary to incise abscess for drainage. After rupture and incise the abscess, it is advisable to use Ba'er Dan or Jiuyi Dan to promote pus discharge and expel the decayed substances, and put medicated paper threads into the incision to enhance the pus coming out, and apply Jinhuang Gao on the infected areas. When pus is discharged completely, it is suggested to apply Shengji San to promote the healing of wound.

1. 2. 2
Breast Mass

It refers to benign hyperplasia diseases of mammary glands, neither inflammation nor tumour, called hyperplasia of lobule of mammary glands in western medicine.

【Diagnosis】

This disease often happens among the women at the age of 25~45, accompanied by distending pain in the breasts. It is usually aggravates before menstruation and relieved after menstruation, closely related to the fluctuation of emotion. The mass can be in the bilateral or unilateral breast, mostly in the upper quadrant or scattered in the whole breast, mass are in soft or slight tough nature, manifested by unclear margin, smooth surface, and good motion and mostly accompanied by tenderness.

【Treatment】

Internal treatment: Syndrome of the accumulation of phlegm due to stagnation of liver Qi, Modified Xiaoyao Loubei San can be applied; Syndrome of the dysfunction of thoroughfare vessel and conception vessel, Modified Er'xian Tang plus Siwu Tang.

External treatment: Application method, it is advisable to apply Yanghe Jiening Gao mixed with Heituixiao Xiao or Guishe San externally on the infected area; or giant typhonium rhizome and fresh pieces of Toad Skin, or rhubarb powder mixed with vinegar, all of above is ok.

1. 2. 3
Mammary Tumour

It includes two kinds: benign tumour and malignant tumour, and the breast lump and breast stone are narrated here.
1. 2. 3. 1
Breast lump

Breast lump is the most common benign tumour in the breast. It is called mammary gland fibroadenoma in Western medicine

【Diagnosis】

It mostly develops among young female, manifested by the round or oval mass with the diameter between 0. 5～5cm, the border is clearly, and the mass in tough nature, smooth surface, palpable elastic sensation. The movable mass often can be touched, and grows slowly, and it enlarges rapidly in the pregnancy period, and should be got rid of the possibility of canceration.

B type ultrasonic wave and molybdenum palladium X—Ray can be helpful to the diagnosis.

【Treatment】

Internal treatment: For Qi of the liver stagnation syndrome, Xiaoyao San can be applied; for blood stasis and phlegm accumulation, modified Xiaoyao San plus Siwu Tang can be applied; if menstruation is not normal, it should be given treatment for thoroughfare vessel and conception vessel.

External treatment: Application Method: It is advisable to apply Yanghe Jiening Gao plus Heituixiao on external local area, and change the dressing once a week.

Other therapies: Generally surgical therapy should be performed to cut it off, and then carry on pathological examinations.

1. 2. 3. 2

Breast Stone

Breast stone is the malignant tumour of breast, also called breast cancer in western medicine.

【Diagnosis】

It often happens in the age of 40~60, especially in the ladies during menopause.

It can be divided into generally type breast cancer and special type breast cancer.

General type breast cancer

It generally has lump with no pain, the border is clear, and firm and hard lump with poorly delineated margins, uneven surface, often fixed to local skin, and sign of dimple in the centre of the local area, fewer accompanied by nipple discharge.

Then with the enlargement of the tumour, different degree pain can develop, oedema as if the orange husk and redness of the skin, nipple retraction or raises, sometimes small erosions, when tumour transmit to axillary and supraclavicular areas, enlarged lymph node can be palpated. When the tumour moves to the armpit and swollen lymph node can be touched.

Special type breast cancer includes that inflammation cancer and eczematoid cancer, etc, and the molybdenum target X—Ray photo, B type ultrasonic wave can aid the diagnosis, and biopsy can diagnose the disease.

【Treatment】

Early diagnosis of breast stone is the key point. In principle, surgical treatment is the most important. The traditional Chinese medicine use mostly in late stage of patients, especially has very good effect on patients after surgeon and can eliminate the poison and increase effect of chemotherapy and radiotherapy, and can raise patient's existence quality, or lengthens existence phase.

Internal treatment: Syndrome of accumulation of phlegm due to stagnation of liver Qi, Modified Shenxiao Gualou San plus Kaiyu San ; syndrome of the dysfunction of Thoroughfare Vessel and conception Vessel, Modified Er'xian Tang plus Kaiyu San ; syndrome of Body deficiency and Toxin hyperactivity, Modified Bazhen Tang; Syndrome of deficiency of Qi and Blood, Modified Renshen Yangrong Tang ; syndrome of deficiency of spleen and stomach, modified Shenling Baizhu San or Lizhong Tang; except above, it is seen that syndrome of deficiency of yin of stomach after chemotherapy and radiotherapy with decayed mouth and bleeding gum, modified Yiwei Tang is administrated to nourish the Yin of stomach.

External treatment: It is suitable for patients that can't be given surgical operation, or the distance extensively shift's patients is not suitable for surgical operation, it is initial stage, using Awei Xiaopi Gao externally and apply it on the breast, after ulcerated, using Haifu San or Bingshi San and Hongyou Gao externally on the breast, and after dropping of the necrosis tissue, apply Shengji Yuhong Gao and Sheng ji San externally on the breast.

Other therapies: Surgical treatment, chemotherapy, endocrine therapy and radiotherapy can be performed, and also, the herbal medicine, Xihuang Wan, Xingxiao Wan and xiao Jin Dan can also be administrated.

1. 3
Wart

Wart is the generic name of thyroid gland disease. It is characterized by happening in the thyroid gland, swelling lumps, or agglomerating, burning pain, mostly unchangeable colour for the local skin. The lump can move with swallowing, or accompanied by tired heat, palpitation, too much sweat and abnormal menstruation, even amenorrhoea, etc. It includes simple goitre, thyroid adenoma, thyroid cyst, thyroid carcinoma, thyroiditis and hyperthyroidism etc.

1. 3. 1
Meat Wart (or exophthalmic goiter)

It is one kind of more common diseases of the wart. The clinical characteristics are Adam's apple on one side or two sides agglomerate before the neck, which is soft, tough and round and like meat mass, and can move with swallowing, and develop slowly. It often happens in young female and middle-aged people. It also can be called thyroid Adenoma or cyst in western medicine.

【Diagnosis】

There are one or two agglomerations in the centre of Adam's apple, and it can move with swallowing. It has semicircle shape and smooth surface, and no painful feeling when be touched, and grows slowly. Usually, it has no general symptoms. Some patients are accompanied by the syndrome of hyperthyroidism, and few can become canceration.

Ultrasonic waves and radioiodine scanning can aid the diagnosis.

【Treatment】

Internal treatment: Qi-stagnation and phlegm-accumulation syndrome can be treated by modified Xiaoyao San plus Haizao Yuhu Tang; Qi and Yin deficiency syndrome can be treated by modified Shenmai San plus Haizao Yuhu Tang.

External treatment: It is advisable to choose Yanghe Jiening Gao mixed Heituixiao or Guishe San to apply to the area externally.

Other therapies: Acupuncture and surgical treatment can be used

1. 3. 2
Lapis Wart (Thyroid Carcinoma)

It is solidly like stone, cannot be moved, and also called thyroid carcinoma in Western medicine.

【Diagnosis】

The patient has swelling lump before neck, which is hard and tough with uneven surface. It can't move when be pushed, and limited movement when swallowing. If it spreads into neck plexus nerve, the patient will have severe pain in the ears, rest head and shoulders; if the lump enlarges, it can cause larynx shift or spreads into throat nerve, the difficulty of breath or swallow will develop. The swelling lymph nodes are sometimes palpable.

Using isotope 131 iodine scanning, B type ultrasonic wave, CT and pathological checking can help to diagnoses.

【Treatment】

Internal treatment: Syndrome of accumulation of phlegm and blood stasis can be treated with modified Haizao Yuhu Tang plus Taohong Siwu Tang. Syndrome of deficiency of Yin and blood stasis can be treated with modified Tongqiao Huoxue Tang.

External treatment: It is advisable to choose Yanghe Jiening Gao mixed Awei San to apply to the areas or raw pokeberry root to painful and burning lump externally.

Other Therapy: After diagnosed definitely, surgical treatment or local radiotherapy should be performed as soon as possible.

1.4
Tumour (Liuyan)

Liu is agglomeration produced by blood stasis, phlegm retention, and turbid qi staying in the tissue of the body. It equals to part of benign tumour on the body surface in modern medicine.

Yan is a general name for the malignant tumour on the body surface, which is the most dangerous one in the surgical diseases. It is hard in quality, uneven in surface, like the stone, so the name is Yan(stone in Chinese). It equals to malignant tumour in the body surface in modern medicine.

In this chapter, the Liu and Yan will be discussed together. And five representative diseases of Liu and Yan are expounded especially; they are blood tumour, fleshy tumour, cocoon lips, cervical carcinoma, and flower-like kidney carcinoma.

1. 4. 1
Blood Tumour

Blood tumour means a kind of tumour due to expansion and being crowd together in length and breadth of superficial venules. It equals to nagioma in modern medicine. The popular blood tumors are capillary angiomas and cavernous hemangiomas.

【Diagnosis】

Capillary angioma, usually on the face and neck of the children, is manifested by red papules or small erythema in the skin, which are expanding gradually, the border of them are clear, the sizes of them are not equal, the quality is soft and they can be compressed, the colour of them is bright red or amaranth, the colour can disappear when pressing, and appear when lifting the hand.

Cavernous hemangioma is manifested by soft quality like sponge, bulge usually with circumscribed hemisphere shape, thin and flat shape, or protrusion above the skin surface. The tumour has great compressibility, it can be engorged by downward sagging position, or shrinks by lifting the diseased limb. The granulo-phlebolith sclerosis can be felt inside the tumour. The trauma can result in bleeding and secondary infection, and the chronic bleeding ulcer may be developed.

【Treatment】

Internal treatment: the virulent fire syndrome of hear and

kidney is treated by modified Qinlian Ermu Wan plus Liangxue Dihuang Tang; the prosperous fire of liver channel syndrome is treated by modified Danzhi Xiaoyao San plus Qinggan Luhui Wan; the spleen loosing controlling function is treated by modified Shunqi Guipi Wan.

External treatment: the small size capillary angioma and cavernous hemangioma are treated by anointing Wumiao Shuixian Gao externally; applying Qingliang Gao plus Tenghuang Gao externally, and then bending up and fixing them; if the tumour is bleeding, the Yunnan Baiyao could be added to it for applying.

Other therapies: injection treatment, the hardened place is injected by Xiaozhiling injection plus 1% procaine in proportion of 1 : 1; the other therapies are operation therapy, cryotherapy, and radiation therapy.

1. 4. 2
Cocoon Lips

Cocoon lips got the name because the shape of it like silk cocoon, it equals to cheilocarcinoma in modern medicine.

【Diagnosis】

The onset of this disease is slow, it is often seen in old male, the local of the disease is often in the juncture of middle 1/3 and outside 1/3 in the red marginal part of the lower lip, it is seldom seen in the corner of the mouth and upper lip. This disease often occurs on the basis of the benign tumors, such as the cornification and hyperplasia, leukasmus, chap, or papilloma that cannot be cured after long time treatment. At the beginning of the disease, the sclerosis is circumscribed, like a bean, and then it increases gradually. There is usually no pain at the beginning, and then the tumour develops into diabrosis like a flower, with untimely bleeding with water, accompanied with pain, and difficulty in opening mouth and taking food. If the condition is aggravated, the patients will have swelling and fixed submandibular and submental lymphnodes, this is usually a sign of cancer metastasis.

【Treatment】

Internal treatment: the fire flaming of heart and spleen syndrome is treated with modified Qingliang Ganlu Yin; the excessive heat of spleen and stomach is treated with modified Liangge San plus Qingwei San; the deficient yin causing excessive fever syndrome is treated by modified Zhibai Dihuang Tang.

External treatment: the tumour is applied with Pi'aijing externally, every day or every other day; the diseased place is applied with Chansu Wan plus vinegar after grinding.

Other therapies: it is treated by taking patent herbs orally such as Xihuang Wan, Xiaojin Pian; in modern medicine, it is treated by operation, radiation therapy, chemical therapy, laser therapy.

1. 4. 3
Cervical Carcinoma

Cervical is tumour in the vertical part or before or behind the ears, it got the name because at the advanced stage of the disease, the qi and blood is deficient, the complexion is pinched, the structure is emaciated like withered leaves and branches of the tree, there is no luster. It equals to cervical lymph nody metastasis and primary malignant tumour in modern medicine.

【Diagnosis】

The cervical carcinoma is manifested by lymphadenectasis in the neck, the tumor develops fast, the quality of it is hard. At the beginning of the disease, it is often singular nodus that can move; at the advanced stage of the disease, the size and the number of the tumours increase, they amalgamate into conglomeration or link into string, the surface is uneven, they are fixed. After a long time, the tumour is broken, there is bloody water seeping from the sore, and the surface is uneven like a flower. The sphere of the swelling and pain may spread to face, chest, shoulder and back.

Overall and meticulous medical check-up and finding the primary lesion or making pathological test of the living tissues are helpful for making final diagnosis.

【Treatment】

Internal treatment: the stagnation of liver qi and coagulation of phlegm syndrome at the initial stage is treated by Kaiyu San; at the middle stage of the stage, the toxin is accumulated and the healthy qi is weak, it is treated by modified Heying Sanjian Wan; at the advanced stage, the qi and blood are wane, it is treated by Xiangbei Yangrong Tang.

External treatment: it is applied with Awei Huapi Gao externally at the initial stage; it is applied with Shengji Yuhong Gao mixed with Hairu San externally after breaking.

Other therapies: it can be treated by taking patent herbs orally such as Xihuang Wan; the local pathological changes are treated by radiation therapy or combining with general chemo, or operation therapy.

1. 4. 4
Kidney Carcinoma

In TCM, penis belongs to the kidney. It equals to carcinoma of penis in modern medicine.

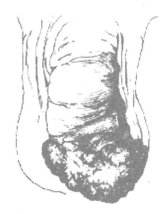

Figure 5   Kidney Carcinoma

【Diagnosis】

This disease is often occurring in middle aged and old people. At the initial stage of the disease, there are papule, erythema, nodus, verrucous hyperplasia etc. near frenulum of prepuce, head of the penis, coronary furrow, or urethral orifice. They could increase gradually, there is pricking and itching feeling, and even they are broken. In the serious cases, the penis is broken and broken off. There is metastasis of the lymphonodes in the local place. There are usually no obvious general symptoms at the initial stage, at the advanced stage, the fever, emaciation, anemia will occur.

The pathological section test can aid the final diagnosis.

【Treatment】

Internal treatment: the accumulated turbid dampness syndrome is treated by modified Sanmiao Wan plus Sanzhong Kuijian Tang; flaming of fire toxin syndrome is treated by modified Longdan Xiegan Tang plus Simiao Yong'an Tang; yin deficiency causing excessive fire syndrome is treated by modified Zhibai Dihuang Wan plus Dabuyin Wan.

External therapies: ① if the tumour is broken and dirty, the Wuwu Dan or Qianjin San are scattered on the wounds, or the tumour is applied with Honglingdan Yougao externally. After the tumour is eroded to even and normal, the medicine is changed to Jiuyi Dan. If the wound is bleeding, the Haifu San may be added, it is applied with Shengji Yuhong Gao externally. After clearing the wounds, the medicine is changed to Hongyou Gao or Baiyu Gao. ② it is applied with Pi'aijing externally, every day or every other day. ③ the diseased place is anointed by flurouracil Gao, 2 times daily.

Other therapies: chemo, radiation therapy, local excision of penis, excision of part of penis, or total excision of penis by operation.

1. 5
Anorectal Diseases

It refers to happen in the perianal and perirectal disease, including that, anal, anal fissure, anal abscess, anal fistula, rectocele, polypus hemorrhoid etc. All of that was called anal hemorrhoid, anal fistula in the traditional books.

1. 5. 1
Hemorrhoid

Hemorrhoid refers to a soft venous ball formed by dilation and varicosis of the rectal venous plexus below the mucous membrane of the rectal end and below the skin of the anal canal.

【Diagnosis】

Main manifestations are painless hematochezia, hemorrhoid coming out of the anus in defecation, wet sensation around the anus and pruritus or swelling and pain in hemorrhoid.

Internal hemorrhoid is what occurs above the dentate line, formed by a plexus of superior hemorrhoidal veins that are covered by mucosa. It can be divided into three phases due to the prolapse of internal hemorrhoid.

External hemorrhoid is what occurs below the dentate line,

formed by venous plexus in lower part of rectum, which covered by skin of the perianal region. It includes thrombotic external hemorrhoid; varicose external hemorrhoid; external hemorrhoid of connective tissue; and inflammatory external hemorrhoid etc.

Mixed hemorrhoid is caused by varicosis and convergence of external and internal hemorrhoids with the symptoms of both external and internal hemorrhoids. Hemorrhoidal mass can come out of the anus in defecation and form a round hemorrhoid and incarcerated hemorrhoid.

【Treatment】

Internal treatment: It is suitable for internal hemorrhoid at the stage of Ⅰ and Ⅱ, or incarcerated hemorrhoid infection or internal hemorrhoid accompanied by other serious chronic diseases is not suitable for surgical therapy.

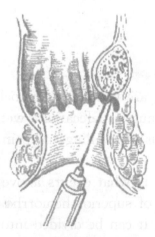

Figure 6   Injection Therapy for Internal Hemorrhoid

Syndrome of blood heat and intestinal Dryness can be treated by modified Liangxue Dihuang Tang, if accompanied by constipation, Runchang Tang is added; syndrome of downward transmission of dampness and heat can be treated by modified Zanglian Wan. Syndrome of Qi stagnation and blood stasis can be treated with modified Zhitong Rushen Tang; syndrome of insufficiency of Gastrospleenic Qi, Modified Buzhong Yiqi Tang can be administrated, if accompanied by blood insufficiency, Siwu Tang is added.

External treatment: It is suitable for various internal hemorrhoid or incarcerated hemorrhoid with swelling and pain. Fumigation and irrigation method are usually employed, and the commonly used herbal drugs are Galla Chinensis, Radix Sophorae flavescentis, etc. Application method: it is advisable to choose Xiaozhi Gao or Wubeizi San for external application. Herb inserting method: after herbal drugs are made into suppository, it is advisable to insert it into the rectum, such as Zhichuang Shuan.

Other therapies: Inserting methods: an effective measure in Chinese medicine treatments. It is to mix the herbal San and sticky nice and then add water to make drug bar with double tips, then insert it into hemorrhoidal nucleus. Then non bacterial inflammatory reaction and hyperplasia of fibre tissue or kraurosis will develop, so as to enhance the hemorrhoid shrinking or casting. Injecting Method: the injecting contents are the hardening-atrophic agent and withering-necrotic agent. Ligation Method: Silk thread penetrating ligation method and rubber ring ligation method are currently employed. Surgical therapy: It includes pure surgical removal, surgical removal for cutting a shuttle incision, and surgical removal for separation of thrombotic external hemorrhoid.

1. 5. 2
Anal Abscesses

The anal abscess refers to the formation of abscess due to a-cute or chronic infection around the anus and rectum, which is corresponding to anorectal abscess in modern medicine.

【Diagnosis】

It happens more in male than in female, especially young and strong male with the main manifestation of pain and external swelling around anus, and accompanied by general symptoms, such as different level fever and tiredness, etc.

Owing to the differences of parts and depth of the abscess, the symptoms also vary. If the abscess is above the anus muscle, the sites is deep and the general symptoms are severe, but localized pain may be slight; otherwise, the general symptoms are slight but localized pain may be severe, such as obviously redness, swelling, heat and aches.

【Treatment】

Mostly, surgical treatments are employed, and meanwhile, and prevent the formation of anal fistula.

Internal treatment: Syndrome of accumulation of heat toxin modified Xianfang Huoming Tang and Huanglian Jiedu Tang; Syndrome of excessive fire-toxins, modified Tounong San; Syndrome of deficiency of Yin and Toxin Lingering, modified Qinghao Biejia Tang plus Sanmiao Wan.

External treatment: In the early stage, it is advisable to choose golden yellow Gao and Huanglian Gao for external application. If the site is deep, golden yellow Gao mixed with water can be applied to clean anal canal rectum. Syndrome of deficiency can be treated with Chonghe Gao or Yanghe Jiening Tang for external application. After the pus is formed, surgery should be employed to enhance the discharge of the pus, and select different surgical ways for different position and degree of abscess. After the pus is discharged, apply cloth thread with Jiuyi San to drainage it. When the pus has discharged completely, it is advisable to use cloth thread Shengji San. If the disease is delayed and formed into anal fistula, it can be treated according to the therapy for anal fistula.

1.5.3
Anal Fistula

The anal fistula refers to rectum or anus opening to the skin and forming into fistula.

【Diagnosis】

A few pus, bloody and mucous secretion can be seen outside the anal fistula. And because the stimulation caused by them, wet sensation or pruritus around the anus, and sometimes eczema will develop. The external opening can be seen in the anus, and the internal opening can be found with a probe.

It can be divided into low simple, low complex, high simple

and high complex anal fistula.

X-Ray and lipiodolography can show the path and depth of the anal fistula, ramification and position of internal opening, relations to round anorectal viscera, and to provide the reliable evidences for surgical operation.

【Treatment】

Internal treatment: Syndrome of downward transmission of dampness and heat can be treated with modified Ermiao Wan plus Bixie Shenshi Tang; syndrome of deficiency of body and toxin Lingering can be treated by modified Tuoli Xiaodu Tang; syndrome of deficiency of body liquid can be treated by modified Qinghao Biejia Tang.

Other therapies: The surgical operation gives first place to therapy. Cut the fistula open totally, sometimes it is necessary to cue off the hard scar tissue along the border of ulcer in order to maintain a smooth drainage and make pus come our easily, and enhance the healing of wound. It is the key for surgical success to correctly find the internal opening and cut it off or incise it, otherwise the wound couldn't be healed and will recur even temporarily healing. Surgical methods are as follows: thread-drawing method, incision method, and the combination of thread-drawing and incision method, etc.

1. 5. 4
Anal Fissure

It refers to an inflammatory disease caused by ulceration due to dehiscence of the whole layer of skin at the anal canal.

【Diagnosis】

Clinically, it is manifested as periodical pain and hemorrhage in the anus, and constipation.

Early anal fissure is manifested by shallow wound, fresh red colour, and smooth border and in soft and elastic nature; Old anal fissure is manifested by long time, repeated attack and progressive pale ulceration, deep bottom, thickened border in a Jar Mouth shape, flat and hard gray-white tissue formed on the bottom. Because of the chronic inflammation in the peripheral tissue of the fissure, it is often accompanied with external hemorrhoid of connective tissue (nickname sentinel pile), internal blind fistula, hypertrophy of anal papilla, a-nal sinusitis, anal papillitis, and etc.

【Treatment】

Internal treatment: Traditional ways can be employed for early treatment; and surgery should be applied to old anal fissure. Syndrome of blood heat and intestinal dryness can be treated with modified Liangxue Dihuang Tang plus Piyue Maren Wan. Syndrome of Yin Deficiency and Fluid Loss can be treated with modified Runchang Tang. Syndrome of Qi stagnation and blood stasis can be treated with modified Liu-mo Tang plus safflower , peach seed, red peony root, and etc.

External treatment: It is suitable for early anal fissure, it is advisable to cover wound with gauze prepared with Shengji

Yuhong Gao ; or to use 1 ∶ 5000 potassium permanganate solution for sitting bath and also Kushen Tang or salt water of peppertree (hua jiao) for sitting bath; For old anal fissure, it is advisable to apply Qisan Dan or Kuzhi San on the wound, after the decay is exfoliated two to three days later, it is advisable to use Shengji San and Shengji Baiyu Gao to heal the wound, or use Changqiang (Du1) occlusive therapy.

Other therapies; For those patients failed non-surgical treatment of old anal fissure or early anal fissure, it is advisable to choose proper surgical methods in accordance with different situation ① Anal dilation method; ② Incision method; ③ Unilateral anal Fissurectomy; ④ Vertical incision and transverse suture.

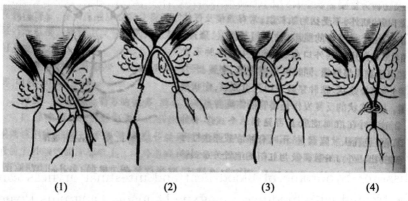

(1)   (2)   (3)   (4)

Figure 7 Tread-drawing Therapy for Anal Fistula

1. 6
Urinary And Male Diseases

It includes urine system and productive system diseases.

1. 6. 1
Male Sterility

It refers to the condition in which a married couple, who lived together more than 2 years with normal sexual life and not taking any contraception measures, finds it difficult to produce an offspring. The defect is with the male partner, but not with the female partner.

【Diagnosis】

The diagnosis should be considered from following points:

The history of disease should be known, and from his past history, marriage history, individual life history, we can find the cause of disease. Based on physic examination, we can know his nutrition and development, and determine whether there has spermophlebectasia.

The laboratory examinations include examination of sperm, testis biopsy and reproductive endocrine determine and genetics test, etc.

【Treatment】

Internal treatment: Syndrome of deficiency of kidney yang can be treated with modified Jingui Shenqi Wan plus Wuzi Yanzong Wan or Yanggaowan Tang. Syndrome of Deficiency of Kidney Yin can be treated with Modified Zuogui Wan plus Wuzi Yanzong Wan. Syndrome of deficiency of Yin and Fire Hyper-activity can be treated with modified Zhibai Dihuang Tang. Syndrome of accumulation and stagnation of liver Qi can be treated with modified Chaihu Shugan San plus Wuzi Yanzong Wan. Syndrome of downward transmission of dampness and heat can be treated with modified Chengshi Bixie Fenqing Tang. Syndrome of Deficiency of Qi and Blood can be treated with modified Shiquan Dabu Tang.

1. 6. 2
Chronic Prostatitis

It is a commonly and frequently disease among the young and middle aged males. In accordance with the clinical features, it can be divided into acute and chronic, or bacterial and non-bacterial, or specific and non-specific prostatitis. The chronic and non-bacterial, non-specific are the most common.

【Diagnosis】

The main clinical manifestations in chronic prostatitis are frequent and precipitant urination, dribbling urination, insidious pain and discomfort in the perineum, and urethral dribbling of white prostatic fluid, simultaneously accompanied by burning and itching sensation in the urethra. Most patients have swelling and painful sensation around pudendum. Long-time disease can cause impotence, premature ejaculation , seminal emission, painful ejaculation, or dizziness, tinnitus,dream-disturbed sleep, and tired waist, etc.

In the digital rectal examination, normal prostate can be palpated with slight tenderness in chronic prostatitis, uneven surface, tough nature, and sometimes slight hypertrophy. The prostate can shrink and turn hard.

Prostatic secretions can aid diagnosis.

【Treatment】

It is suggested to treat the patients systematically and impor-
tance should be attached to the care. Clinically, the majority
is treatment based on syndrome differentiation, and the
three basic pathological links, i. e. , kidney deficiency (foun-
dation), dampness and heat (indication), stagnation (variation) should be identified, and the drugs should be administrated correspondingly.

Internal treatment: Syndrome of heat-toxin accumulation can
be treated with modified Bazheng San or Longdan Xiegan
Tang; Syndrome of Qi stagnation and Blood stasis should be
treated with modified ceianliexian Tang. Syndrome of Yin
deficiency and excessive fire-evil should be treated with modified Zhibai Dihuang Tang, and syndrome of deficiency of
kidney yang can be treated with modified Jisheng Shengqi
Wan.

External treatment: Take a sitting bath with Conggui
Tazhong Tang for 20 minutes each time, twice a day. Insert
Yejuhua Shuan or Qianlie Shuan into the rectum about 3～
4cm, twice a day.

Other therapy: It is necessary to choose antibiotics sensitive
to pathogenic bacteria. As for physical therapy, local super-
shortwave heat therapy or local effective antibiotic ion penetrating therapy can be employed.

1. 6. 3
Prostatic Hyperplasia

Prostatic Hyperplasia is also called prostatic enlargement, and it is one of the most commonly encountered diseases in the old males in the clinical urinary surgery.

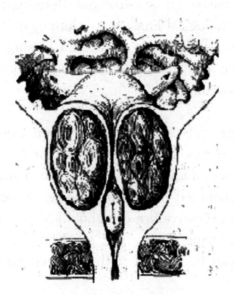

Figure 8   Prostatic Hyperplasia

【Diagnosis】

It occurs often in the males over 55 years old, characterized mainly by frequent and urgent urination, difficult urination, and even dysuria, and dribbling urine. It is highly possible to induce acute retention of urine for cold, tired, retention urine, and constipation, even lead to renal damage. Some patients can have complications such as urine infection, vesical calculus, hernia and rectocele.

In digital rectal examination, bilateral lobes of the prostate are enlarged, symmetrically, in an elasticity, smooth surface, and shallow or disappeared central groove. Type B ultrasonic examination, CT, dynamic examination of urine, bladder urethrocystography, cystoscope can aid diagnosis.

【Treatment】

Warming and replenishing kidney-yang or resolving stasis and promoting urination are the basic therapeutic rules. Chinese traditional medicine and modern medicine should be used when accompanied with complications.

Internal treatment: Syndrome of downward transmission of dampness and heat can be treated with modified Bazheng San. Kidney yin deficiency syndrome can be treated with Zhibai Dihuang Wan; Kidney Yang syndrome can be treated with modified Jisheng Shenqi Wan. Syndrome of Qi stagnation and blood stasis can be treated with modified Chenxiang San. Syndrome of deficiency of kidney and spleen can be treated with modified Buzhong Yiqi Tang plus dodder seed, desertliving cistanche, malay tea scurfpea fruit, plantain seed etc.

External treatment: Application of herbal medicine externally or clyster treatment can be employed, and if necessary, catheterization can be applied.

Surgery, medicine treatment, physical and acupuncture treatment can also be applied.

1. 7
Peripheral Vascular Disease

Peripheral vascular disease is the vascular disease which excluding cardiovascular and cerebrovascular system. It can be divided into arteriosis and phlebocholosis. Arteriosis include thromboangiitis obliterans, arteriosclerotic obliteration, arterial embolism, multiple takayasu arteritis, aneurysm etc and disorders of peripheral arterial relaxation and contraction such as Raynaud's disease, erythematous acrodynia and so on. Phlebocholosis include Thrombotic superficial phlebitis, thrombosis of deep vein, valvular disorder of deep vein, varicosity etc.

Peripheral vascular disease is named as vascular disease by Chinese medicine for peripheral vessels are itemized as meridian or vessels.

1. 7. 1
Shank Sore

Shank Sore is chronic ulcer of skin on the shin bone of shank often as anaphase complications of fascial sarcoma. In western medicine it is named as chronic ulcer of lower extremity.

【Diagnosis】

This disease is commonly seen in the long standers and rower, often as one of anaphase complications of fascial sarcoma.

At the beginning shank is swelling with a heavy sensitivity and local venous engorgement. Then a series of intravenous malfunction such as superficial phlebitis, pigmentation, congestive dermatitis and eczema gradually happen following lasting swelling on the internal and outer edge of lower part of legs and crack, infiltration and ulceration on the skin of lichen appearance. In the anaphase sore begins to cave in with margin up as the orifice of jar, surface grey and dirty, infiltration and the circumference deeply red or violet, or eczema and itching, hard to recover. When secondary infection happens, the ulcer can suppurate or cause to hemorrhage. Some critical cases' ulcer can expand to much part of blow knee and dorsum and reach to periosteum. A few patients can get carcinomatous change for unrecovering in many years.

The test of venous valve's function of lower extremity can help to verdict the function of valve. Angiography of veins of lower extremity and ultrasound Doppler test of blood stream can assist to diagnosis.

【Treatment】

Internal treatment: Moist heat downward syndrome can be treated with modified Simiao Wan and Wushen Tang; the syndrome of weakness of Qi and obstruction of blood can have modified Buyang Huanwu Tang.

External treatment: in the initial stage, those whose local is red and swelling and much infiltration should be washed with the decocted traditional Chinese medicine. Those whose local skin has little infiltration can be covered with Jinghuang Gao. In the anaphase, stall the adjusted Qiceng Dan mixed with sesame oil on the surface of sore and bind it with binder. When slough is exfoliated and new flesh is exposed, Shengji San is covered with Shengji Yuhong Gao. Qingdai San mixed with sesame oil can be pasted on the skin with eczema.

Other treatments: In western medicine, ulcer of leg mainly is taken with operation, local therapy, wearing elastic socks and so on.

1.7.2
Gangrene

Gangrene, also named Tuo Gu Ju, is a kind of chronic peripheral vascular disease on all extremities, in severity dactylopodite gangrene is dropped. It is just like Buerger disease, arteriosclerosis emphraxis and the bad foot of diabetes mellitus.

【Diagnosis】

Buerger disease is commonly found among young male, especially on lower extremities with the history of coldness, wetness, smoke, trauma and so on. Arteriosclerosis emphraxis, often among aged man, accompany with hyperlipemia, hypertension, arteriosclerosis, damaging big and medium-sized artery. The bad foot of diabetes mellitus is a part of diabetes mellitus, damaging big and medium-sized artery.

According to the process of the disease, three phases are clinically classified as ischemia phase, dystrophy phase, and necrosis phase or putrefaction phase.

Ultrasound Doppler of extremities, graph of blood stream, microcirculation of nails, arteriography and blood fat and sugar can help to clear diagnosis and differential diagnosis and comprehend the severity of cases.

【Treatment】

The only Chinese medicine or western medicine can be use to the early phase of this disease, the combined therapy of traditional Chinese and western medicine to the severity. The Traditional Chinese medicine thinks highly of syndrome differentiation and treatment, mainly promoting blood circulation and removing blood stasis along all the process. The drugs are injected to build up collateral circulation and ameliorate blood circulation.

Internal treatment: The syndrome of veins occlusion with coldness and dampness is treated with modified Yanghe Tang; the syndrome of blood stasis with modified Taohong Siwu Tang; The syndrome of poison of dampness and heat with modified Simiao Yongan Tang; the syndrome of damage of Yin of heat and poison with modified Gubu Tang; the deficiency syndromes of Qi and Yin with modified Huangqi Biejia Jian. These syndromes should be added Maodongqing Jian and injection of tanshinone. According to etiological factor, the drugs to lower blood fat and blood pressure should be used to the patients with arteriosclerosis emphraxis and the measure of control blood sugar, regulate therapy and anti-infection can improve the status of the patients with the bad foot of diabetes mellitus and recover blood circulation.

External treatment: The undefeated sore can be treated with Chonghe Gao and Hongling Danyou Gao; Cover Shengji Yuhong Gao when sore is open and little; When sore is large and necrosis constitution is hard to drop, first use borneo camphor and Zinc oxygen oil to soften the induration, then according to the degree of softness, delete necrosis crust by turns, soft tissues and then rotten bone. The thorough debridement can be carried out after inflammation disappears, or perform amputation.

1.8
Other Surgical Diseases

Other Surgical Diseases involve chilblain, burn, and bite by insect or beasts, tetanus and enteron sore and so on. This chapter introduces burn.

Burn

Burn is a kind of local or general impairment caused by heating power (such as flame caloric gas, liquid or solid), electric energy, chemistry, radiation.

【Diagnosis】

The depth of burn has a common classification of three degrees and four levels, degree I, degree II, (light II and deep II), degree III.

The classification of the degree of severity, to design good treatment program, divides burn into four degree: minor burn, moderate [degree] burn, deep burn, and the most serious burn.

【Treatment】

Internal treatment: The syndrome of saliva damage by heat and poison is treated with Huanglian Jiedu Tang, Yinhua Gancao Tang, Xijiao Dihuang Tang or Qingying Tang; the syndrome of deficiency of both Yin and Yang with Sini Tang, modified Shenfu Tang and Shengmai San; the invagination syndrome of heat and poison with Qingying Tang or modified Huanglian Jiedu Tang and Xijiao Dihuang Tang; the syndrome of delirium, add Angong Niuhuang Wan or Zixue Dan; the syndrome of weakness of Qi and obstruction of blood, with Tuoli Xiaodu San or Bazhen Tang added to honeysuckle flower, Mongolian milkvetch root ; the syndrome of insufficiency of spleen and damage of Yin, with modified Yiwei Tang and Shenling Baizhu Tang.

External treatment:

(1) Locally clear wound on the basis of preventing and treating shock.

(2) The initial stage: the little degree Ⅰ, degree Ⅱ, should be covered Jingwanhong empyrosis ointment, Qingliang Gao, Zicao Gao, Wanhua You, without binding; Or compress with sesame oil mixed powder of garden burnet root powder and rhubarb powder, changing on every other day.

Larger burn of degree Ⅱ without skin damage,

should be spurted Hudi Ding a few times every day; Clear out the damaging skin and smear with Shirun Shaoshang Gao.

Burn of degree Ⅲ should be compressed with intensity of magnetism to keep dry and to prevent infection. Those who have good status, should be cut crust and operate skingrafting or protect crust and operate skingrafting; Shuihuo Tangshang Gao and Chuangzhuo Gao can be used to drop crust.

(3) Metaphase: The surface of damage is infected, so some drugs and methods can be taken according to the surface and the infectivity. Huanglian Gao, Hongyou Gao, Shengji Yuhong Gao can be compressed on the little area of infection; Those big area of infection with much water should compress wetly with 2% coptis liquid, 2% amur amur corktree liquid, 10% giant knotweed rhizome. When crust includes empyema, to uncover and drain as soon as possible, then soak or wet compress with the above-mentioned liquid. Otherwise select the responding drugs according to the test of pus bacteria cultivation and drugs' sensitivity.

(4) Anaphase: When rotten fresh drop and newly born fresh product, compress Shengji Baiyu Gao, Shengji Yuhong Gao and Shenji San.

Other treatments: Including first aid at site and therapy with western medicine.

1.9

Dermatosis And Sexual Transmitted Disease

Dermatosis is the disease on skin, mucosa and skin auxiliary. Sexual transmitted disease, also named venereal disease, is a lot communicable disease infected through sexual touch, similar sexual behavior and indirect contact.

1.9.1
Tinea

Tinea is a superficial fungal dermatosis attacking epidermis, hair or nails. This chapter only discusses several common fungal dermatosis, like tinea capitis, tinea manus and pedis, tinea corporis, etc.

【Diagnosis】

Clinic manifestation

Tinea capitis is similar to Tinea blanca in western medicine. It is capable of a natural cure when the patient reaches adolescence, and the baldness can get regeneration. No scar will be left after recovery.

Tinea favosa is similar to yellow ringworm in western medicine. Later, the hair follicles become damaged, resulting in permanent trichomadesis.

Tinea unguium is similar to tinea manus in western medicine. Its skin eruption is characterized by vesicle on the centre of palm or between the fingers. Keratoderma, desquamation and vesicle on the palm are all possible. After relapses, palm skin gets thickening, withered, painful and difficult to bow or stretch. It turns into tinea unguium when attacking nails.

Tinea pedis is similar to foot tinea in western medicine. It has vesicle type, erosive type and desquamation type. The skin lesion is common in first two types.

Tinea circinata is similar to tinea corporis in western medicine. Its skin lesion is circular or multicircular shape with obvious edges. The center of plaque extincts with its surrounding dilated. It gives a feeling of itching and may get lichenoid change after too much scratching.

Pityriasis simplex on the face is similar to tinea versicolour in western medicine. The skin lesion can be light brown, gray brown, heavy brown, little depigmentation or with chaff-like scales. It is recurrent.

2. Laboratory examination: Eumycetes direct microscopic examination, eumycetes cultivation and evaluation. Deep mycosis needs tissue pathologic examination.

【Treatment】

The chief principle is killing parasites to relieve itching and it should be treated thoroughly. Antifungal which should be applied has certain advantages. External treatment is the main method for tinea. If the skin lesion is extensive, or self-conscious symptoms are severe, or improper scratching causes infection, it should be combined with internal treatment.

Internal treatment: The syndrome of wind-damp-toxin is treated with Xiaofeng San; the syndrome of damp-heat downward flow with the majority of dampness is treated with Bixie Shenshi Tang; the syndrome of damp-heat with blood stasis is treated by Wushen Tang; the syndrome of e-qual damp-heat with Longdan Xiegan Tang.

External treatment: No. 1 Xianyaoshui, No. 2 Xianyaoshui, 3% boracic acid solutions, Erfan Tang can be chosen for tin-ea according to different condition. 60g Cardinal can be boiled into a decoction to immerse attacked skin for 15 minutes. Pizhi Gao or Xionghuang Gao can be externally applied.

Other treatment: Antifungal like Sporostatin, Itraconazole, Terbinafine can be chosen for oral medication. $5 \sim 10\%$ Brimstone Gao, 50% Propanediol, paraimidazole paracryl-amide cream or solutions can be chosen for externally use.

1.9.2
Damp Sores

A damp sore is allergic and inflammatory dermatosis, which is similar to eczema in western medicine.

【Diagnosis】

(1) Acute damp sores are similar to acute eczema in western medicine.

The onset is abrupt. Its skin lesion appears symmetrically, primarily and is polymorph including erythema, flush skin, papular eruption, vesicles, pustule, exudation, crust, etc. It is capable of attacking any part of the skin, mostly the face, head, posterior auricle, limbs and perineum symmetrically.

(2) Subacute damp sores are similar to subacute eczema in western medicine.

It is often turned into a protracted case when acute eczema has not received timely treatment or has been treated improperly. It also can primarily be subacute. The skin lesion is less severe than that of acute eczema, and mainly appears papular eruption, crust and scales with a few vesicles and mild erosion. There exists a severe itching that becomes more serious at night.

(3) Chronic Damp Sores, similar to chronic eczema in western medicine.

The skin lesion is always limited and appears thick, coarse and hard, dark red or purplish brown, possibly with obvious wrinkles or lichenoid changes. Some skin lesion may contain new papular eruption or vesicles. There exists a severe paroxysmal itching, and it becomes more serious at night especially when patients get nervous, drink alcohol or eat hot food. It has a long course and easy relapse, sometimes severe and sometimes mild.

【Treatment】

The main therapeutic method for eczema is to clear heat, remove dampness and stop itching. For the acute, the main treatment is to clear away heat and remove dampness. For the chronic, the main treatment is to nourish blood and moisturize skin. The drug for external treatment should be mild to avoid worsening patients' condition.

Internal treatment: The syndrome of damp-heat brewing in the skin is treated with modified Longdan Xiegan Tang and Bixie Shenshi Tang; the syndrome of damp-heat infiltration and immersion with modified Longdan Xiegan Tang and Wu-wei Xiaodu Yin; the syndrome of spleen vacuity with damp encumbrance with modified Chushi Weilin Tang or Shenlin Baizhu San; the syndrome of blood vacuity and wind dryness with modified Danggui Yinzi or Siwu Xiaofeng Yin.

External treatment

(1) For acute damp sores, Flavescent Sophora Root (ku shen), Phellodendron Bark (huang bai), belvedere fruit, fineleaf schizonepeta herb can be boiled into a decoction for warm washing; If vesicles have obvious erosions and exudation, amur corktree, Dried garden burnet root, purslare herb, Wild Chrysanthcmum Flowcr can bc boilcd into a decoction for wet packing, then use the mixture of Natural Indigo Powder and Sesame oil as liniment; Subsequently, when there is little exudation, Cop-

tis Root Gao and Natural Indigo Paste can be selected for external application.

(2) For subacute damp sores, the principle of external treatment is to stop inflammation and itching, to dry and astringe exudation. Sanhuang, 3% Unguentum Picis Fabae Nigrae, 10% Dried Sanguisorba Root Zinc Oxide Oil can be selected for external application.

(3) For chronic damp sores, Natural Indigo Paste, 5% Sulfur Gao, 5%~10% Compound Pine Tar Gao can be selected for external application.

Other treatment: Antihistaminic, Sedative, Vitamin can be chosen in western medicine. Zinc Oxide Oil, Boric Acid Lotion, Glucocorticoid Powder can be selected for external application.

1. 9. 3
Psoriasis

Psoriasis is a chronic itchy dermatosis characterized by thickening and hardening of the skin that gives it the appearance of the skin of an ox's neck, similar to neurodermatitis in western medicine.

【Diagnosis】

It tends to occur on the neck and frontal part; other possible parts include the sacrococcygeal region, the cubital fossa, and the popliteal fossa. It can also occur on lumbus, back, hips, vulva, perianal part, groin and limbs. Its skin lesion appears symmetrically, or follows skin wrinkle and cutaneous nerve.

The skin lesion starts with the appearance of flat papules that tend to gather, in normal skin colour or light brown with luster. Gradually, the local skin extends, gets dry and thick with little desquamation, and forming lichenoid patches with dermal ridges and deepened stripes after scratch. The patient has intense paroxysmal itching, especially at night or in emotional variation

The localized: The skin lesion, localized on neck and nape, takes the form of lichenoid changes or thickened skin with clear edges.

The Universal: The skin lesion is wide-ranging, mostly on the cubital fossa, the popliteal fossa, limbs, face, and trunk and capable of attacking any part of the skin.

This disease has a protracted and recurrent course.

【Treatment】

The principle of treatment is dispersing wind to clear heat, enriching the blood and moistening dryness. For secondary infection, antimicrobial needs to be applied.

Internal treatment: The syndrome of fire involving liver meridian is treated with modified Longdan Xiegan Tang; the syndrome of wind-damp brewing in the skin with modified Xiaofeng San; the syndrome of blood vacuity and wind dryness with modified Danggui Yinzi.

External treatment: For syndromes of fire involving liver meridian and wind-damp brewing in the skin, Three Huang Lotion can be selected for external application. For blood vacuity and wind dryness syndrome, heating Gao for torre-faction can be used; Yangtigen San mixed with vinegar can be externally applied once or twice daily.

Other treatments: Acupuncture, plum-blossom needle and acupoint injection can be applied.

1. 9. 4
White Crust

White Crust is a recurrent inflammatory dermatosis, similar to psoriasis in western medicine. The name comes from symptoms: the skin is itchy and white like pine bark after scratch.

【Diagnosis】

(1)Clinic manifestations

White Crust tends to attack young people, especially male sex with genetic factors. It attacks the patients or becomes more severe in winter, but less severe in summer. Several years after attacking, this seasonal change is not so obvious.

This disease is clinically classified into four types: the common type, the pus-pocket type, the articular type and the erythroderma type.

(2) Laboratory and other accessory examination

Increase of leukocytes, faster blood sedimentation and negative pus-pocket bacterial culture are common with different manifestation in histopathology examination.

【Treatment】

The common type can be treated with Chinese medicine based on different syndrome and sign; the pus-pocket type, the articular type and the erythroderma type should be treated by the combination of Chinese medicine and western medicine.

Internal treatment: The syndrome of hemopyretic inner brewing is treated with modified Xijiao Dihuang Tang; the syndrome of blood vacuity and wind dryness with modified Danggui Yinzi; the syndrome of qi and blood stagnation with modified Taohong Siwu Tang; the syndrome of damp toxin brewing with modified Bixie Shenshi Tang; the syndrome of excessive fire-toxin with modified Qingwen Baidu Yin.

External treatment: For the skin lesion in progress, the treatment should be mild, like Huanglian Gao, Pulian Gao; For the skin lesion in silent period and regression, dregs of decoctions can be boiled to immerse the attacked skin, then Huanglian Gao can be externally applied.

Other treatment: Antibiotics, Vitamin, immunosuppressant, immunotherapy, venous block therapy and physiother-apy can be chosen in western medicine. Acupuncture, ear acupuncture, pricking and cupping are all effective.

1. 9. 5
Red Butterfly-like Sore

Red Butterfly-like Sore, an autoimmune disease, attacks skin and internal organs, similar to Lupus Erythematosus in western medicine.

【Diagnosis】

1. Clinical manifestation: It is classified into red butterfly-like sore discoides and systemic red butterfly-like sore, with the latter for the majority.

> (1) Discoides red butterfly-like sore attacks mostly fe-males among 20 to 40 years old. The skin lesion tends to occur on the face and may also involve dor-sum manus, the edge of finger, lips and scapular region.

> (2) Systemic red butterfly-like sore mostly attacks young and middle-aged females, ten times as long as males.

> The skin and mucosa lesion has diverse manifesta-tion in early stage with obscure symptoms. It may attack single organ or several systems, manifes-ting fever, arthralgia, myalgia, renal injury, car-diovascular pathologic change, respiratory patho-

logic change, nervous system pathologic change, lymphatic system, hematopoietic system and ocular fundus pathologic change.

2. Laboratory examination: Hemocyte analysis, urinalysis, immunologic examination is helpful for diagnosis.

【Treatment】

The treatment in Chinese medicine is to tonify liver and kidney, activate blood circulation and dissipate blood stasis, expel wind by detoxification. It is usually combined with western medicine in clinic.

Internal treatment: The syndrome of noxious heat should be treated with Xijiao Dihuang Tang and Huanglian Jiedu Tang; the syndrome of deficiency of Yin and excessive heat with modified Liuwei Dihuang Wan and Dabuyin Wan, Qinggu San; the syndrome of spleen and kidney Yang deficiency with modified Fugui Bawei Wan and Zhenwu Tang; the syndrome of spleen deficiency due to liver hyperactivity with modified Sijunzi Tang and Danzhi Xiaoyao San; the syndrome of Qi-stagnation and blood stasis with modified Xiaoyao San and Xuefu Zhuyu Tang.

External treatment: Apply Baiyu Gao and Huangbo Shuang onto the sore, once or twice one day.

Other treatment: Corticosteroid hormone, immunosuppressant may be chosen in western medicine for acute attack or severe cases. Chinese patent medicine like tripterygium hypoglaucum hutch tablet, common threewingnut root multig-

lycoside tablet, sweet worm extract tablet, compound Jin-
qiao tablet can be chosen for oral administration.

1. 9. 6
Syphilis

Syphilis is a chronic contagious venereal disease caused by
the spirochete treponema pallidum, possible to attack the
whole body. It can be grouped under the category of "Mei-
chuang","Ganchuang","Hualiubing" in Chinese medicine.

【Diagnosis】

According to Clinic manifestation, history of dirty coitus or
sexual spouse with syphilis history can help diagnosis.

Primary syphilis has the manifestation of chancre, local
lymphadenectasis; second syphilis has the manifestation of
syphilitic lesions, skin and mucosa lesion, injury of bones,
ocular syphilis, nerve syphilis, etc; third syphilis, also
called late syphilis, attacks several organs besides skin and
mucosa lesion.

Incubatory syphilis, also called latent syphilis, has no clinical manifestation with normal cerebrospinal fluid. Serum reaction is positive and other diseases that may cause it can be
eliminated.

1. Congenital syphilis: Treponema pallidum in mother's
blood infects fetus through placenta. It can heavily influence
baby's health with severe organ injury, and its case-fatality
rate is high.

2. Laboratory examination: positive treponema pallidum antigen serum test, positive treponema pallidum ribonucleic acid in polymerase chain reaction, or treponema pallidum found in tissue secretion is confirmed diagnosis for syphilis.

【Treatment】

Penicillin, tetracycline or erythromycin is the primary choice for syphilis and Chinese herb is accessory treatment.

Internal treatment: The syndrome of damp-heat in liver meridian can be treated with Longdan Xiegan Tang plus glabrous greenbrier rhizome, giant knotweed rhizome; the syndrome of toxin brewing with hemopyrexia with modified Qingying Tang and Taohong Siwu Tang; the syndrome of Toxin in tendon and bones with modified Wuhu Tang; the syndrome of deficiency of liver and kidney with modified Dihuang Yinzi; the syndrome of deficiency of heart and kidney with modified Linggui Zhugan Tang.

External treatment: For gan sore, apply Ehuang San or Pearl powder on the attacked skin. When skin with bubo sore and late syphilis is not inflamed, cover the mixture of Chonghe Gao and equal vinegar and alcohol on the lesion; When inflamed, cover Wuwu Dan first and then Yuhong Gao on the surface of sore; After rotten flesh and pus disappear, put Shengji San in the sore and cover Hongyu Gao. The red bayberry sore can be washed with the decoction of wild Tuckahoe (tu fu ling), common cnidium fruit (she chuang zi), pepper of Sichuan (chuan jiao), dandelion (pu gong ying), radish seed (lai fu zi) and densefruit pittany root-bark (bai xian pi).

1.9.7
AIDS

AIDS is an acronym for Acquired Immune Deficiency Syndrome, which is infected with the Human Immunodeficiency Virus (HIV). Its manifestation is according to pestilence, consumptive disease, scrofula, mass in the abdomen in Chinese medicine.

【Diagnosis】

Clinical manifestation: It has incubation period from six months to five years or longer. The disease has three phases: infected phase, phase of relative syndrome, and phase of AIDS syndrome according to the degree of cellular immunity deficiency.

Immune test: test of HIV and the HIV antibody can help to clear diagnosis.

【Treatment】

There is no specific remedy to AIDS. The immunomodulator, antivirus drug and complex treatment can control the development of AIDS, elongate the survival time and enhance the quality of life. The Chinese medicine and other natural treatment have much practice for preventing and treating AIDS. Many herbs have selected to treat some patients for their function of defending HIV virus and enhancing body immunity, which should be guided by differential usage. In the same time, acupuncture and moxibustion have a good function in the treatment for its all-round regulation.

1. Syndrome differentiation and treatment: The syndrome of lung damage by pathogenic factors can be treated with modified Yinqiao San or Jingfang Baidu San; The syndrome of the Yin weakness of lung and kidney with Baihe Gujin Tang and Gualou Beimu Tang added to giant knotweed rhizome, Common selfheal fruit-spike, nepal dock root etc; the syndrome of weakness of spleen and stomach, with Buzhong Yiqi Tang and Shenling Baizhu San add to glubrous greenbrier rhizome, Tianjihuang, Miaozhuacao etc; the sufficiency of spleen and kidney, with Shenqi Wan and Sishen Wan added to chuling and radix glycyrrhizia etc; the syndrome of weakness of Qi and stasis of blood, with Buyang Huanwu Tang, Xijiao Dihuang Tang and Xiaolei Wan; The syndrome of phlegm turbidity in Yang orifices with Angong Niuhuang Wan, Zixue Dan, Zhibao Dan. If more coldness, use Suhexiang Wan to remove phlegm and then use Shenmai San to reinforce Qi and Yin.

2. Some common effective herb and expectant treatment

(1) Effective herbs of antivirus: radix glycyrrhizia, ginseng , dangshen, astragalus root, largehead atractylodes rhizome, Indian bread, Chinese angelica, jujube, barbary wolfberry fruit, eucommia bark, epimedium, lightyellow sophora root, bupleurum root, manypricklc acanthopanax root, mushroom, dan shen root, golden thread, honeysuckle flower, baical skullcap root, snakegourd root, tokyo violet herb, etc.

(2) Herbs of enhancing phagocytic function of mononu-
clear leukocyte: herba Epimedii, slenderstyle acanthopanax bark, largehead atractylodes rhizome, solomonseal rhizome, mythic fungus, dandelion, honeysuckle flower, danshen Root, peach seed, red
peony root, chuanxiong rhizome, mushroom, poria
from Yunnan of China, liquorice etc.

(3) Herbs of enhancing phagocytic function of macro-
phage: mythic fungus, chuling, mushroom, Chinese
angelica, rehmammia root, Indian bread with hostwood, herba Epimedii, malytea scurfpea fruit,
manyprickle acanthopanax root, eucommia bark
etc.

(4) Herbs of adding T cells: largehead atractylodes rhizome, coix seed, solomonseal rhizome, cochinchi-
nese as paragus root, glossy privet fruit, herba epimedii, etc.

(5) Herbs of improving cellular immunity: donkey-hide
Gelatin, dodder seed, herba epimedii , ecliptae,
Chinese Angelica, safflower, hairyvein agrimonia
herb, danshen Root, rehmammia dried rhizome,
glossy privet fruit, wolfberry fruit, white peony
root, chuanxiong rhizome, honeysuchle flower,
golden thread etc.

(6) Herbs of improving immunity of body fruit: dansh-
en root, safflower, chuanxiong rhizome, Chinese
Angelica, hairyvein agrimonia herb, rehmannia

dried rhizome, glossy privet fruit, wolfberry fuit, white peony root, honeysuchle flower, Chinese magnolivine fruit etc.

(7) Herbs of elongating survival of antibody and stimu-lating production of HIV antibody: dwarf lilyturf tuber, figwort root, root of seraight ladybell, fresh-water turtle shell, suberect spatholobus, donkey-hide gelatin, glossy privet fruit, etc.

(8) Herbs of elongating survival of antibody: cassia bark, prepared lateral root of aconite, common curculigo rhizome, herba epimedii, songaroa cyno-morium herb, dodder seed, they can stimulate the output of antibody and the transformation of lym-phocyte.

Chapter 2 Osteology And Traumatology

The osteology and traumatology of Traditional Chinese Medicine (TCM) is a subject that directed by the theory of TCM, and aim to study, prevent and treat bone, joint and adjacent soft tissue injury. Mainly contents include two parts: injury and bone disease. Injury is composed of fracture, dislocation, soft tissue injury and injured internal syndrome, what induced mainly by external force hurt, invasion by six exogenous pathogens or pathogenic toxicity and internal deficiency of vital qi. There are extensive contents in bone disease, including congenital osteomalformation, osteocarbuncle, bone and joint tuberculosis, bone and joint paralysis syndrome, malnourished syndrome, soft tissue spasm, bone and joint degenerative disease, osteochondral disease, metabolic bone disease, bone tumour, etc. Bone disease is often the result of congenital deficiency of kidney essence, postnatal insufficiency of primordial qi, skeleton vacuity, and invasion by pathogenic toxicity.

2. 1
Fracture

A fracture is the destruction of the continuity and integrality of a bone when undergoing external force and the clinical symptoms mainly include the followings: local pain, swelling, loss of function, acute progress, abnormal movement and bony crepitus, etc. Fracture is a common multiple and injury disease in clinic. In the past long run, treated fractures with TCM has produced systematic theory and accumulated abundant clinical diagnostic and therapeutic experiences, especially in the way of reduction manipulation, splint fixation, exercises of function and TCM therapy, with significant effects.

【Etiology and Pathogenesis】

It is possible to get a fracture when an external force is placed upon human body, such as direct excessive force, indirect excessive force, extreme muscle contraction or chronic strain, etc. Fracture fragments can displace, there are five patterns in fracture displacement: angled displacement, lateral displacement, shorten displacement, separated displacement and rotated displacement, these often be seen at the same time in clinic.

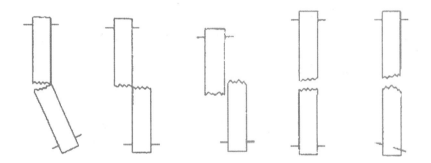

Figure 9   Five patterns in fracture displacement

Classifications of fracture: ① According to whether wound in skin communicates with fracture: closed fracture and open fracture. ② According to various injury degrees: simple fracture, compound fracture, incomplete fracture and complete fracture. ③ According to the shape of fracture line: transverse fracture, oblique fracture, spiral fracture, comminuted fracture, impacted fracture, compressed fracture,

linear fracture, greenstick fracture and separation of the e-
piphysis. ④ According to the stability after fracture reduction: stable fracture and unstable fracture. ⑤ According to
the time of fracture: fresh fracture and stale fracture. ⑥
According to whether the bone matter is normal or not:
traumatic fracture and pathologic fracture.

Complications of fracture: After undergone excessive force,
besides fracture, systemic and local complications are likely
to occur in human body: ① Traumatic shock. ② Infection,
especially open fracture is prone to infection. ③ Viscera injury, include lung, liver and spleen, bladder and urethra injury. ④ Important arterial injury. ⑤ Ischemic muscle
spasm. ⑥ Spinal cord injury. ⑦ Peripheral nerve injury. ⑧
Fat embolism. ⑨ Hypostatic pneumonia. ⑩ Bed sore. ⑪
Infection and calculus of urinary tract. ⑫ Traumatic ossification. ⑬ Traumatic osteoarthritis. ⑭ Joint ankylosis. ⑮
avascular necrosis of bone. ⑯ Tardive malformation. Etc.

【Diagnosis】

Most fractures only result in local symptoms, and severe
fracture and multiple fractures can induce systemic re-
sponse.

Local features

(1) the common features of fracture: local pain, swelling and functional disturbance.

(2) The specific signs of fracture: ① deformity: Fracture fragments' displacements can change the out-

line form of the injured limb, mainly express as shorten, angled or rotated deformity. ②Abnormal movements: There are abnormal movements after fracture in the part that couldn't move before fracture. ③Bony crepitus: After fracture, grating sensation either heard or felt as bone ends rub together.

Bone X-Ray examination: X-Ray examination is important in diagnosis and treatment of fracture. It can reveal the indiscoverable incomplete fracture, deep fracture, intra-articular fracture and little avulsion fracture in clinic.

【Treatment】

The principles of fracture treatment include reduction, fixation and exercises of function.

(1) Reduction, to get the normal or approximately normal anatomic relation of displaced bone ends back and rebuilds the supporting effects of bone. Reduction by manipulation: it is a therapy which doctors' fingers, palm, twist, arm and/or other parts of body are used in combined with instruments, by different manipulations in different fractures, apply in suffered parts and points, to cure disease, treat injury and reduce fracture. The indications of manipulation: injured diseases such as fracture, dislocation and soft tissue injury. The basic reduced manipulation: ① Pull and traction. ② Rotation. ③ Fold and gore. ④ Convolute. ⑤ Uptake and lift.

⑥ Restrain correctly. ⑦ Dispart bones. ⑧ Flexion and extension. ⑨ Longitudinal press.

Open reduction: excide the adjacent soft tissue of fracture in surgery, expose the bone ends, reduce fracture directly.

(2) Fixation, include external fixation and internal fixation. External fixations include splint fixation, plaster cast fixation and continual traction. ① Splint fixation, little splints are made up of flexible willow board, bamboo board or plastic board, add mat in appropriate position, and fix bone ends by tape splints outside limb with straps. The indications of splint fixation: closed fractures in long bones of limbs, for femoral fracture, as the strong strength of femoral muscle, the splint fixation must combined with continual bone traction; open fractures in limbs, with little and cicatrized wound after treatment; stale fractures in limbs that indicated closed reduction. Splint fixation can effectively prevent lateral, rotated or angled displacement, and can remedy the remainder lateral and angled displacement due to the stress of straps and mat; splints are applied to exclude the joint above and below the fracture line, that's useful to early exercises of function, stimulate bone growth and healing and prevent joint ankylosis. Splint fixations possess the advantages of reliable fixation, faster bone healing, good functional rehabilitation and less complications. ② Plaster cast fixation, can be used for open fracture after debridement and suture;

some special position such as vertebral fracture, after some open reduction with a internal fixation operation; after orthopedic operation and limb with osteocarbuncle. ③ Continual traction includes skin traction, cloth bracket traction and bone traction.

(3) Functional exercises can stimulate the systemic and local circulation of qi and blood, harmonize and unify the functions of zang-fu viscera; prevent disused myoatrophy, osteoporosis, joint ankylosis and conglutination of scars; under effective fixed strength, the reduced bone ends are incline to stabilized by the contraction and extension, antagonism, extrusion of muscles; and help to faster functional rehabilitation of limbs. Functional exercises in Osteology and Traumatology give attention to both local and system, combined with stabilization and movement, is an effective method to quicken functional rehabilitation.

2. 2
Dislocation

A dislocation is displacement of a bone end from the joint, there is usually functional disturbance of articular, and the clinical symptoms include local pain, swelling, functional disturbance, joint deformity, vacuity of glenoid cavity and flexible fixation, etc.

【Etiology and Pathogenesis】

The main causes of dislocation are external force and chronic strains, etc.

Classifications of dislocation: ① according to the causes of dislocation: traumatic dislocation, pathologic dislocation and habitual dislocation. ② according to various dislocated degrees: incomplete dislocation and complete dislocation. ③ according to the direction of dislocation: anterior dislocation, posterior dislocation, superior dislocation, inferior dislocation and central dislocation. ④ according to the time that after dislocation: fresh dislocation and stale dislocation. ⑤ according to whether wound in skin communicates with articular cavity: closed dislocation and open dislocation.

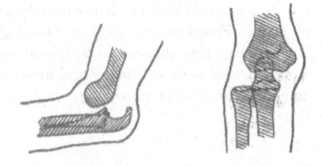

Figure 10　Elbow Joint Posterior Dislocation
Combined with Radialis Dislocation And Deformity

Complications of dislocation: fractures, blood vessels injury, nerves injury, avascular necrosis of bone, traumatic ossification and traumatic osteoarthritis.

【Diagnosis】

It's not difficult to make a diagnosis according to medical history, local swelling, pain, joint deformity, flexible fixation, action disturbance and can touch the vacuity of articular cavity or dislocated articular head, X-Ray examination can ascertain the direction and type of dislocation.

【Treatment】

The treatments of dislocation mainly include reduction with manipulation, fixation, functional exercise and pharmacotherapy.

Manipulations of reduction are composed of pull and traction, flexion and extension, uptake and lift, etc; use different manipulations according to different dislocations. Fixations of dislocation include cloth bracket fixation, bandage fixation and splint fixation. After early reduction, the dislocated joint can move moderately, active exercises of articular function are encouraged after remove the fixation, but the rough motion is forbidden.

The general principle of medicine therapy is promoting blood circulation for removing blood stasis and relieving rigidity of muscles and activating collateral.

2.3
Soft Tissue Injury

Soft tissue injury is the injury of skin, muscles, fascias, tendons, ligaments and cartilages, peripheral nerves and major blood vessels because of twist, contusion, stab, cutting and strain.

【Etiology and Pathogenesis】

Excessive external force, extreme muscle contraction, chronic strain, invasion by six exogenous pathogens or pathogenic toxicity and asthenic body can induce soft tissue injury.

Classifications of soft tissue injury: ① according to the character of injury: twist and contusion. ② according to injury degree: avulsion, rupture and semi-dislocation. ③ according to the course of injury: acute and chronic soft tissue injury. ④ according to if there is wound in skin or mucous membrane: open and closed injury.

Complications of sift tissue injury: avulsion fracture, nerves injury, myositis ossificans, intra-articular dissociative air and osteoarthritis.

【Diagnosis】

With case history of strain, local pain, action disturbance, some with myoatrophy in long course, local sensory disability, local press pain, general after ruling out fracture, dislocation and local infection.

【Treatment】

Soft tissue injury can treated with tendon-soothing maneuver, acupuncture and moxibustion therapy, little needle-knife therapy, traction therapy, physical therapy and pharmacotherapy.

Manipulation commonly used includes superficial Tuina, deep Tuina, kneading, shove collateral, scrape, rolling, beat, pinch, press point, flexion and extension, rotation and wobble, lumbar extension, press and trample, quiver and slub method.

The general principle of medicine therapy is promoting blood circulation for removing blood stasis and relieving rigidity of muscles and activating collateral.

2.4
Injured Internal Syndrome

Injured internal syndrome is dysfunction of Qi and Blood, zang-fu viscera and meridians due to zang-fu viscera being damaged, mainly include injured static blood, injured pain, injured fever, injured abdominal distension, injured fainting, etc.

【Etiology and Pathogenesis】

Injured bleeding occurs when excessive force is placed upon human body, result in channels damaged, and blood spill over vessels. It can be classified in external hemorrhage and internal hemorrhage according to the hemorrhagic position; in ounce bleeding, moderate bleeding and massive bleeding according to the volume of bleeding. The blood extravasation due to blood-heat after injury; it also can induce bleeding from the nine orifices of the five sense organs. Massive bleeding can lead to the syndrome of blood deficiency.

Injured pain is the damage of Qi and Blood as a result of external force hurt human body, qi stagnation or coagulation and stagnation of static blood, stagnation of qi and blood may bring about pain. In general, lumbar twist and contusion often combine with qi stagnation, all kinds of contusion with static blood, other injury both with qi stagnation and static blood. Vital qi is damaged after injury, invasion by exogenous pathogenic factors also result in pain.

Injured fever owing to the stagnation of static blood after injured or fever of the invasion by exogenous pathogenic factors.

Injured abdominal distension is the result of cohesive gastroenteric air after injured, qi stagnation then the symptom of ventral flatulence appears.

【Diagnosis】

The patient has definite traumatic history, injured bleeding, and blood flow from wound or the nine orifices of the five sense organs; when internal bleeding in limbs, the limbs will swell and pain, in the coelom such as thorax and abdomen, thoracoabdominal pain, pale complexion and weakness and disability will appear.

Injured pain shows distensible pain, sting, ache, syndrome of heat transformed from stagnation or infected by pathogenic toxicity will show red, swelling, heat and pain.

Injured fever, fever with static blood usually occurs one day after injury, without chill, sometimes with hematoma. Fever due to infected by pathogenic toxicity is often hyperthermia, with chill, can find the focus of infection. Fever due to blood deficiency usually occurs at afternoon, with the symptom of vertigo.

【Treatment】

Injured bleeding need first aid and hemostasis, supply the blood capacity, saving from the prostration by strengthening qi.

Injured pain can treated with promoting blood circulation to restore qi-movement, dispelling pathogenic wind and cold, clearing heat-toxin methods according to different syndromes.

Injured fever, treatment based on syndrome differentiation, uses promoting blood circulation, removing toxic substance, nourishing blood methods.

Injured abdominal pain, treated with eliminating stagnant blood by catharsis, regulating qi-flowing for activating stagnancy, invigorating spleen and replenishing qi methods according to different syndromes.

Operative treatment: blood vessel ligation, repairing operation, repairing operation of fracted viscera is applicable to those patients with bleeding.

2.5
Bone Disease

There are extensive contents in bone disease, include congenital osteomalformation, osteocarbuncle, bone and joint degenerative disease, osteochondral disease, bone tumour, etc.

【Etiology and Pathogenesis】

(1) Etiology: ① internal causes: the reality of congenital development, age, corporeity, state of nutrition, and functional status of zang-fu viscera, all of these can influence the occurrence of bone disease. ② external causes: invasion by six exogenous pathogens, infected by pathogenic toxicity, chronic strains, regionally factors, poison and radiation will induce bone damage.

(2) Pathogenesis: ① Pathogenesis of external pathogens: invasion of wind pathogen, pain caused by cold pathogen, fire pathogen injuring Yin. ②Pathogenesis of Qi and Blood: Qi stagnation, static blood, Qi deficiency, Blood deficiency concern bone disease. ③Pathogenesis of meridians: meridians obstruction, coagulation and stagnation of Qi and Blood can cause bone disease. ④Pathogenesis of zang-fu viscera: insufficiency of kidney essence, dysfunction of liver in controlling conveyance and dispersion, dysfunction of spleen in transportation, that cause malnutrition of soft tissues and bones, osteomalformation, obstacle of bone metabolism, disorder of joint.

【Diagnosis】

There are many categories about bone disease, with various clinical features. In this section, we just introduce Osteoporosis for an example.

Osteoporosis is common in elders; the mainly clinical features are local pain, deformity and fracture. Pain often located in thoracic and lower lumbar vertebral body. Pain aggravate after ascend and change the body position. With the development of osteoporosis, the compressed vertebral body fracture will occur, with shorten height and gibbous deformity. X-Ray examination will detect decreased bone mineral density (BMD), vertebral bodies were compressed and result in double-concave deformity or wedgy change, cortical bone of cannular bone became thin. Nitrogen and double-photon absorption (DPA) càn detect BMD, which can be used for early diagnosis.

【Treatment】

Medicine therapy: patients with deficiency of spleen qi can be treated with shenling baizhu San and modifications; with deficiency of kidney yin, treat with Zuo Gui Wan and modifications; with deficiency of kidney yang, treat with Zuo Gui Wan and Modifications; with stagnation of Qi movement, treat with Liqi Zhitong Tang. Traditional Chinese patent medicines and simple preparations: Duhuo Jisheng Wan, Jianbu Huqian Wan, Liuwei Dihuang Wan.

External treatment: apply Shangke Xiaoyan Gao, Zhenggu liquid.

Other therapies: calcium, sexual hormone, Vitamin D, fluoride therapy, physical therapy can also be used.

In addition, enhance the exercises of function, pay attention to nutrition of foods.

中医外科 骨伤科
常见病诊疗常识

李乃卿

曹建春

中国中医药出版社

·北 京·

图书在版编目（CIP）数据

中医外科 骨伤科常见病诊疗常识/李乃卿等编著. —北京:中国中医药出版社,2005.12

（中医药对外宣传丛书）

ISBN 7-80156-827-3

Ⅰ.中... Ⅱ.李... Ⅲ.①中医外科—常见病—诊疗—汉、英②中医伤科学—常见病—诊疗—汉、英

Ⅳ.①R26②R274

中国版本图书馆 CIP 数据核字（2005）第 070218 号

中国中医药出版社出版

北京市朝阳区北三环东路 28 号易亨大厦 16 层

邮政编码:100013

传真:(86-10)64405719

北京市松源印刷有限责任公司印刷

各地新华书店经销

*

开本 787×960 1/16 印张 10 字数 114 千字

2005 年 12 月第 1 版 2005 年 12 月第 1 次印刷

*

定价:20.00 元

网址 WWW.CPTCM.COM

总 前 言

中医药是中华民族优秀文化的重要组成部分,几千年来为中华民族的繁衍昌盛做出了不可磨灭的贡献,并且对世界的文明进步产生了积极影响。它是我国卫生事业的重要组成部分和人类医学的宝贵财富。

中医药学是研究人体生命活动变化规律和调节方法的一门科学,体现了对人体生命科学的深刻认识,具有科学性和先进性。中医药学的健康理念和临床医疗模式,体现了现代医学发展趋势。

中医药学拥有一套完整的、独特的理论体系,在临床各科多种疾病的诊疗方面积累了丰富的经验并有确切疗效。作为世界传统医学的优秀代表,中医药对于许多疾病,特别某些现代疑难杂病,如心脑血管病、糖尿病、肿瘤、免疫性疾病、病毒感染性疾病等的诊治,具有独特的优势,正在发挥着越来越重要的作用。

21世纪,随着医学模式的转换,疾病谱发生了变化,医源性、药源性疾病以及老龄性疾病逐渐增多,人们预防保健意识不断增强,国际社会对天然药物的需求日益扩大,中医药的发展必将拥有更加广阔的发展空间,对人类健康事业做出更加巨大的贡献。

为了使中国传统医药在全球发扬光大,传播中医药防治临床各科疾病的科学知识,国家中医药管理局启动了"中国中医药国(境)外传播资料编译系列"项目,这套普及型丛书的编译也是其中的一部分。在此,我们将中医药学科的基础知识介绍给大家,本套丛书共分为12分册,包括中医药学基础、中医药学简史、中医养生保健学、中医药学临床各科、推拿学、针灸学、中药和方剂、中医药国内外发展概况、少数民族医学。本套丛书内容丰富、言简意赅、浅显易懂、生动活泼,图文并茂,有助于国内外读者在较短时间内正确了解中医药的基本知识,熟悉中医药在市场保健和疾病预防方面的应用,以适应现代人对于高品质健康生活的追求。

国家中医药管理局
2005 年 12 月

前　言

我们知道,西医外科学一般以手术或手法为主要疗法,来治疗损伤、感染、肿瘤、畸形,以及其他性质的疾病。那么中医外科和骨伤科治疗什么病呢?

中医外科学的研究范围除了疮疡、乳房疾病、瘿、瘤、岩和皮肤、肛肠、男性前阴、周围血管及其他外伤性疾病外,还包括内痈(如肝痈、肠痈等)、急腹症、疝、泌尿生殖和性传播疾病等。骨伤科包括损伤和骨病。

要想了解中医外科学,就让我们简略回顾一下它的历史吧!

中医外科和骨伤科有着悠久的历史。出土的殷商时期甲骨文已有外科病名的记载。周代(公元前1066~公元前249年),外科已成为独立的专科。《内经》阐述了痈疽疮疡的病因病机,提出用截趾手术治疗脱疽。汉末华佗(141~203年)应用麻沸散作为全身麻醉剂,进行死骨剔除术。南北朝时期,龚庆宣的《刘涓子鬼遗方》(483年)是中国最早的外科学专著,记载了当时处理创伤的情况。隋代,巢元方的《诸病源候论》(610年),记述了断肠缝连,腹疝脱出等手术,采用丝线结扎血管。唐代孙思邈的《千金要方》(652年)书中记述的手法整复下颌关节脱位,与现代医学的手法复位相似;而其用葱管导尿治疗尿潴留的记载,比1860年法国发明橡皮管导尿早1200多年。金元时代,危亦林的《世医得效方》(1337年)记录了正骨前先用乌头、曼陀罗等麻醉;用悬吊复位法治疗脊柱骨折。明代陈实功的《外科正宗》，记述了刎颈切断气管应急用丝线缝合刀口。清代设有治疗骨折和脱臼的专科。

古代治疗疾病的丰富经验在现代有很多发扬、提高。这里也作一简要介绍。

中华人民共和国成立以来，中医外科和骨伤科取得了不少重大进展。在临床方面主要体现在一些特色鲜明、优势明显的专科专病的治疗上，有些科研成果已达到世界先进水平。自20世纪50年代开始，以中医为主的中西医结合防治急腹症得以广泛开展，取得了一定成绩。慢性骨髓炎的中医药和中西医结合治疗取得了显著成绩，尤其对于已形成死骨、骨腔积脓、形成窦道者，疗法独特，治疗效果明确。

乳房疾病方面，中医药治疗浆细胞性乳腺炎、乳晕瘘管、乳腺增生病取得了较大进展。

中医治疗周围血管疾病利用外治与内治的综合优势，必要时与手术、介入疗法并用，取得了较好的疗效。不仅对疾病早期治愈率高，而且对疾病后期的有效率也比较理想，降低了复发率和致残率。

对烧伤的研究主要体现在中药制痂法和湿润暴露疗法的研究方面，同西医处理明显不同。中医治疗肛门痔瘘疾病也取得了较大发展，采用切开挂线法解决了高位肛瘘的难治之点；外剥内扎术是治疗混合痔的改进手术；消痔灵硬化剂注射治疗内痔效果满意。中医诊治尿石症、慢性前列腺炎也有很好的治疗效果。在治疗男性不育症、性功能障碍的临床和试验研究方面，也取得了可喜成绩。

应用中医药治疗恶性肿瘤具有延长生存期、提高生存质量及调整机体免疫功能等作用。中医药配合手术、放疗、化疗,可以促进术后恢复,减轻毒副反应,提高治疗效果。

　　骨伤科工作者在继承传统中医骨伤经验基础上,运用现代科学知识和方法,总结出新的正骨八大手法,研制成功新的夹板外固定器具,同时配合中药内服、外治及传统的功能锻炼方法,形成了一套中西医结合治疗骨折的新疗法,提出了"动静结合"、"筋骨并重"、"内外兼治"、"医患合作"治疗骨折的原则,取得了骨折愈合快、功能恢复好、患者痛苦少及合并症少的良好效果,使骨折治疗提高到一个新的水平。

　　应用中医药治疗皮肤病也取得了可喜的成果,对皮肤真菌病、湿疹、皮炎有较好的临床疗效。在中医药治疗系统性红斑狼疮等结缔组织疾病中,雷公藤制剂的运用对改善症状、调节机体免疫功能均有很好的作用。

　　近年来,从中草药中筛选抗艾滋病毒药物,以期有效地改善艾滋病患者症状,提高生存质,延长生存时间。

李乃卿

目　　录

■■■ 第 1 章　中医外科学 ■■■■■■■■■■■■■■■■■■■■■■■■■■

1.1　疮疡 …………………………………………………… 1

　1.1.1　局部感染 ………………………………………… 1

　1.1.2　全身性感染 ……………………………………… 6

1.2　乳房疾病 ……………………………………………… 8

　1.2.1　乳房感染性疾病 ………………………………… 8

　1.2.2　乳癖 ……………………………………………… 10

　1.2.3　乳房肿瘤 ………………………………………… 11

1.3　瘿 ……………………………………………………… 12

　1.3.1　肉瘿 ……………………………………………… 13

　1.3.2　石瘿 ……………………………………………… 13

1.4　瘤岩 …………………………………………………… 14

　1.4.1　血瘤 ……………………………………………… 15

　1.4.2　茧唇 ……………………………………………… 16

　1.4.3　失荣 ……………………………………………… 16

　1.4.4　肾岩 ……………………………………………… 17

1.5　肛门直肠疾病 ………………………………………… 18

　1.5.1　痔 ………………………………………………… 19

　1.5.2　肛痈 ……………………………………………… 20

　1.5.3　肛漏 ……………………………………………… 21

　1.5.4　肛裂 ……………………………………………… 23

1.6　泌尿男性疾病 ………………………………………… 24

　1.6.1　男性不育 ………………………………………… 24

　1.6.2　慢性前列腺 ……………………………………… 24

　　1.6.3　前列腺增生症 ………………………………… 26

1.7　周围血管病 ……………………………………………… 27

　　1.7.1　臁疮 ………………………………………………… 27

　　1.7.2　脱疽 ………………………………………………… 28

1.8　其他外科疾病 …………………………………………… 30

1.9　皮肤及性传播疾病 ……………………………………… 31

　　1.9.1　癣 …………………………………………………… 31

　　1.9.2　湿疮 ………………………………………………… 33

　　1.9.3　牛皮癣 ……………………………………………… 34

　　1.9.4　白疕 ………………………………………………… 35

　　1.9.5　红蝴蝶疮 …………………………………………… 36

　　1.9.6　梅毒 ………………………………………………… 38

　　1.9.7　艾滋病 ……………………………………………… 39

第 2 章　骨伤科学

2.1　骨折 ……………………………………………………… 42

2.2　脱位 ……………………………………………………… 45

2.3　筋伤 ……………………………………………………… 47

2.4　损伤内证 ………………………………………………… 48

2.5　骨病 ……………………………………………………… 49

第 1 章 中医外科学

1.1 疮疡

疮疡是各种致病因素侵袭人体后引起的体表化脓性疾患,与现代外科感染性疾病类似,可以分为全身性感染和局部感染,局部感染性疾病主要有疖、痈、发、疔疮、丹毒、红丝疔、疽、流注、瘰疬、流痰等;全身性感染则包括走黄和内陷。

就让我们来看一看它们有哪些临床表现和治疗方法。

1.1.1 局部感染

1.1.1.1 疖、痈、发、有头疽

【诊断】

疖、痈、发、有头疽都是发于体表的急性化脓性疾病,大都有局部红肿热痛的临床特点。疖,中西医病名相同;痈,相当于西医的皮肤浅表脓肿、急性化脓性淋巴结炎等,它的特点是局部光软无头,结块范围在 6~9 cm 之间;发,相当于西医的蜂窝组织炎,多在身体疏松部位突然红肿蔓延成片,灼热疼痛,伴有明显全身症状;有头疽,相当于西医的痈,多在皮肤韧厚部位发生,范围多超过 9cm。这些疾病按照病情演变均可分为初起、成脓和溃后三个阶段,初起表现为局部红肿热痛和功能障碍;成脓则局部肿势高突,疼痛加剧,痛如鸡啄,按之中软应指,为脓已成;溃后流脓,实证多脓出稠厚黄

白色,虚证则脓液稀薄,疮面新肉不生。

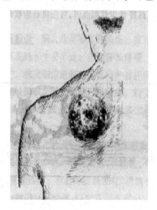
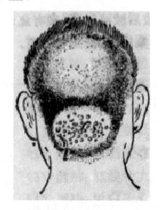

图 1　背部痈　　　　　　　　图 2　项部有头疽

【治疗】

内治　①初起宜疏风清热、解毒利湿,治疗以仙方活命饮等方加减治疗。壮热口渴者加生石膏、天花粉;痉厥加安宫牛黄丸或紫雪丹。②成脓若脓出迟缓者,宜透脓,用透脓散。③溃后脓泄过多,宜补益气血,血虚用四物汤,气虚用四君子汤,气血两虚用八珍汤。

外治　①初起,宜清热消肿,用金黄散、玉露散外敷,或用千捶膏、太乙膏掺红灵丹或阳毒内消散外贴。②成脓,宜切开排脓。③溃后,初宜提脓祛腐,用八二丹或九一丹,并用药线引流;脓尽宜生肌收敛,以生肌散掺入疮口中,并用太乙膏和生肌玉红膏盖贴。

总之,凡是有局部红肿热痛的浅表化脓性疾病均可参照此法治疗。

1.1.1.2　颜面部疔疮

本病是指发生在颜面部位的急性化脓性疾病,相当于西医的颜面部疖、痈。其特征是疮形如粟,坚硬根深,如钉钉之状。头面部为诸阳之会,火毒蕴结,易于走黄,引起生命危险。

【诊断】

初期:开始在颜面部出现粟米样脓头,或痒或麻,以后逐渐红肿热痛,肿势范围多在 3～6cm,但多根深坚硬,形如钉钉之状,重者有恶寒发热等症状。

中期:发病后 5～7 天之间,肿势逐渐扩大,四周浸润明显,疼痛加剧,脓头破溃。伴有发热口渴,便干溲赤,舌红苔黄腻,脉象弦滑数等症状。

后期:约 7～10 天间,肿势局限,顶高根软溃脓,脓栓随脓外泄,肿消痛止,身热减退,一般 10～14 天可痊愈,为顺证。相反,凡颜面部疔疮,特别是生在鼻翼、上唇部的疔疮,可因妄加挤压,不慎碰伤,过早切开等,引起顶陷色黑无脓,周围皮色暗红,肿势扩散,失去护场,以致头面五官俱肿。伴有壮热烦躁,神昏谵语,乃疔毒走散,是为走黄。

【治疗】

内治　清热泻火、凉血解毒,以五味消毒饮、黄连解毒汤、犀角地黄汤加减治疗。

外治　初起宜箍毒消肿,用金黄散、玉露散或千捶膏敷贴,或用六神丸、紫金锭研碎醋调外敷;脓成宜提脓祛腐,用九一丹、八二丹撒于疮顶部,再用玉露膏或千捶膏盖贴。若脓出不畅,用药线引流;若脓已成熟,中央已软有波动感时,应及时切开排脓;溃后宜提脓祛腐,生肌收口,疮口掺九一丹,外敷金黄膏;脓尽改用生肌散、太乙膏或红油膏盖贴。

1.1.1.3　丹毒、红丝疔

为皮肤突然发红,色如涂丹的一种急性感染性疾病,中西医学均称为丹毒。红丝疔是发于四肢,皮肤红丝显露,迅速向上走窜的急性感染性疾病,相当于西医的淋巴管炎。

【诊断】

丹毒多发于小腿、颜面部。初起往往先有恶寒发热、头痛骨楚。继则局部皮肤见小片红斑,迅速蔓延成大片鲜红斑,边界清楚,略高出皮肤表面,压之皮肤红色减退,放手后立即恢复。病情严重者,红肿处可伴发紫癜、瘀点、瘀斑、水疱或血疱,偶有化脓或皮肤坏死。

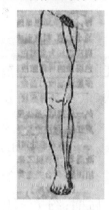

图3 下肢红丝疔

红丝疔好发于四肢内侧,常有手足部生疔或皮肤破损等病史。多先在手足生疔部位或皮肤破损处见红肿热痛,继则在前臂或小腿内侧皮肤上起红丝一条或多条,迅速向躯干方向走窜,上肢可停于肘部或腋部,下肢可停于腘窝或胯间。腋窝或腘窝、腹股沟部常有瘰核肿大作痛。

【治疗】

内治 宜凉血清热解毒。发于头面部的用普济消毒饮加减;发于胸腹腰胯者,用龙胆泻肝汤加减或化斑解毒汤加减;发于下肢者,用五神汤合萆薢渗湿汤加减;赤游丹或毒邪内攻,用犀角地黄汤和黄连解毒汤加减。

外治 外敷金黄散或玉露散;用七星针或三棱针叩刺患部皮肤或红丝疔部位,放血泄毒,外敷太乙膏掺红灵丹。

1.1.1.4 无头疽

无头疽是发生于骨与关节间的急性化脓性疾病的统称。本处只介绍附骨疽和环跳疽,相当于西医的化脓性骨髓炎、化脓性髋关节炎。

【诊断】

附骨疽：初起肢痛彻骨，继则皮肤微红微热，胖肿骨胀，病变的骨端有深压痛和叩击痛；3～4周后成脓；溃后，脓出初稠后稀，淋漓不尽，不易收口，形成窦道，探查可触及死骨。

环跳疽：表现为髋部筋骨疼痛，活动受限；继则疼痛肿胀加剧，有些可触及波动感，全身高热不退；溃后排出脓液，因已损骨，不易愈合，可致关节畸形、僵硬，或造成脱位而致残废。

锝－MDP、[67]镓骨显像对本病的早期诊断有帮助。X线摄片、CT检查、局部穿刺有助于诊断。

【治疗】

内治　初起，清热化湿，行瘀通络，用黄连解毒汤合五神汤加减；成脓，清热化湿，和营托毒，黄连解毒汤合仙方活命饮加减；溃后，调补气血，清化余毒，用八珍汤合六味地黄丸加减。

外治　初起，用金黄膏或玉露膏外敷，患肢或关节用夹板或石膏固定；成脓，宜早期切开排脓；溃后，用七三丹或八二丹药线引流，红油膏或冲和膏盖贴，有骨坏死者应清除死骨，形成窦道者，用千金散或五五丹药线腐蚀扩大疮口，再用药线引流，或作清创术。

1.1.1.5　瘰疬、流痰

瘰疬是一种发生于颈部的慢性化脓性疾病。流痰是一种发于骨与关节间的慢性化脓性疾病。因其可随痰流窜于病变附近或较远的组织间隙，壅阻而形成脓肿，破损后脓液稀薄如痰。

【诊断】

瘰疬:初期颈部淋巴结肿大,质韧,边界不清,渐渐增大,皮核粘连,有时互相融合成块。后期,切开或自溃后,脓水清稀,夹有败絮样物,疮口呈潜行性空腔,疮面肉色灰白,四周皮肤紫暗,可形成窦道。

流痰:常有其他部位的痨病史,以肺痨多见。病变部位以脊椎最多,其次为下肢髋、膝、踝关节,再次为上肢肩、肘、腕关节等。本病初起关节疼痛,伴功能障碍;中期,关节肿胀明显,周围肌肉萎缩,在病变附近或较远处形成脓肿;溃后流脓清稀,夹有败絮样物质,久则疮口凹陷,周围皮色紫暗,形成瘘管不易收口。脓液培养可有结核杆菌生长。必要时可取病灶组织做病理检查有助于明确诊断。

【治疗】

内治　气滞痰凝证以开郁散加减;阴虚火旺证以六味地黄丸合清骨散加减;气血两虚证以香贝养荣汤加减。

外治　初期,局部肿块处可敷冲和膏或用阳和解凝膏掺黑退消,5～7日一换。中期,外敷冲和膏,如脓成未熟,改用千捶膏。脓熟宜切开排脓,创口宜大,或作十字切口,以充分引流。后期,已溃者一般先用五五丹提脓祛腐,脓尽用生肌散收口。如有空腔或窦道时,可用千金散药线,也可用扩创或挂线手术。

1.1.2　全身性感染

1.1.2.1　走黄

走黄与内陷为疮疡阳证疾病过程中,因火毒炽盛,或正气不足,导致毒邪走散,内攻脏腑的危险证候。相当于西医的全身性急性化脓性疾病。继发于疔疮的常称为走黄;除疔以外的其他疮疡引起者称为内陷。

【诊断】

走黄,多有疔疮病史,局部症状一般多为在原发病灶处忽然疮顶陷黑无脓,肿势软漫,迅速向周围扩散,边界不清,失去护场,皮色转为暗红。全身症状有寒战、高热、头痛、烦躁、胸闷,或伴恶心、呕吐、腹泻;或咳嗽、气喘、痰血;或身发瘀斑,风疹块,黄疸等;甚至出现神志昏迷等。

【治疗】

内治　五味消毒饮、黄连解毒汤、犀角地黄汤三方合并加减。神识昏糊,加紫雪丹或安宫牛黄丸;咳吐痰血,加象贝母、天花粉;咳喘,另加鲜竹沥;大便秘结,苔黄腻,脉滑数有力,加生大黄(后下)、元明粉(分冲);痉厥,加钩藤、龙齿、茯神;并发黄疸,加生大黄(后下)、生山栀、茵陈。

外治　疮顶陷黑处用八二丹,盖以金黄膏,四周用金黄散或玉露散冷开水调制以箍围,并时时湿润。其他参照原发疔疮外治法。

其他疗法　早期应用大剂量广谱抗生素;维持水、电解质平衡及对症处理;清开灵 40ml,稀释后静脉滴注,每日一次。

1.1.2.2　内陷

内陷为疮疡阳证疾患过程中,因正气内虚,火毒炽盛,导致毒邪走散,正不胜邪,毒不外泄,反陷入里,客于营血,内传脏腑的一种危急疾病。因多由有头疽患者并发,故名疽毒内陷。根据病变不同阶段的临床表现分为三种:火陷、干陷、虚陷。

【诊断】

多见于老年人，或以往有消渴病史者。局部症状为疮顶不高或陷下，肿势平塌，散漫不聚，疮色紫滞或晦黯，疮面脓少或干枯无脓，脓水灰薄或偶带绿色，腐肉虽脱而疮面忽变光白板亮，新肉难生，局部灼热剧痛或不痛。

全身症状有高热寒战，或体温不升，头痛烦躁，或精神不振，甚至神昏谵语，气粗喘急；或气息低微，胸闷胸痛，咳嗽痰血，恶心呕吐，腹胀腹痛，便秘或腹泻，多汗肢冷，或痉厥，或黄疸等。

一般而言，火陷辨证为邪盛热极证；干陷辨证为正虚邪盛证；虚陷辨证为脾肾阳衰证或阴伤胃败证。

【治疗】

须中西医结合综合救治。

内治　邪盛热极证，以清营汤合黄连解毒汤、安宫牛黄丸或紫雪散加减；正虚邪盛证以托里消毒散、安宫牛黄丸加减；脾肾阳衰证，以附子理中汤加减；阴伤胃败证，以益胃汤加减。

外治　可以参照"有头疽"。

其他疗法可参照"走黄"处理。

1.2　乳房疾病

1.2.1　乳房感染性疾病

乳房感染性疾病包括非特异性感染和特异性感染。非特异性感染可分为乳痈、乳发等；特异性感染主要是乳痨；各种感染治疗不当可发生乳漏。本处介绍乳痈。

乳痈

乳痈是由热毒入侵乳房而引起的急性化脓性疾病。相当于西医的急性化脓性乳腺炎。

【诊断】

多见于哺乳期妇女。初起，乳房局部肿胀疼痛，皮色不变，皮肤不热或微热。或伴有全身不适，恶寒发热，食欲不振，脉滑数。成脓，患乳肿块逐渐增大，局部疼痛加重，或有雀啄样疼痛，皮色焮红，皮肤灼热，同侧腋窝淋巴结肿大。肿块中央渐渐变软，按之应指有波动感，穿刺抽吸有脓液，全身症状加剧。溃后，可破溃出脓，或手术切开排脓，肿消痛减，寒热渐退，疮口逐渐愈合。

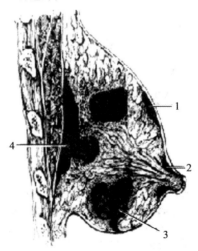

1. 表浅脓肿 2. 乳晕下脓种
3. 深部脓肿 4. 乳房后脓肿

图 4 乳痈

血常规检查可有白细胞总数及中性粒细胞数增加。超声检查有助于深部脓肿的诊断。

【治疗】

内治　气滞热壅证,乳汁郁积结块,肿胀疼痛,以瓜蒌牛蒡汤加减;热毒炽盛证,乳房肿痛,皮肤焮红灼热,以透脓散加味;正虚毒恋证,溃脓后乳房肿痛虽轻,但疮口脓水不断,脓汁清稀,愈合缓慢或形成乳漏,以托里消毒散加减。

外治　初起,可用热敷加乳房按摩,促进郁滞的乳汁排出。可用金黄散或玉露散外敷,或用六神丸研细末,适量凡士林调敷。成脓,应在波动感及压痛最明显处及时切开排脓。溃后,用八二丹或九一丹提脓拔毒,并用药线插入切口内引流,切口周围外敷金黄膏。待脓净仅有黄稠滋水时,改用生肌散收口。

1.2.2　乳癖

乳癖是乳腺组织的既非炎症也非肿瘤的良性增生性疾病。相当于西医的乳腺增生病。

【诊断】

多发生在 25～45 岁。乳房胀痛,常在月经前加剧,经后疼痛减轻,或疼痛随情绪波动而变化。乳房肿块可发生于单侧或双侧,大多位于乳房的外上象限,也可见于其他象限。肿块的质地中等或质硬不坚,表面光滑或颗粒状,活动度好,大多伴有压痛。

【治疗】

内治　肝郁痰凝证,以逍遥蒌贝散加减;冲任失调证,以二仙汤合四物汤加减。

外治　用阳和解凝膏掺黑退消或桂麝散局部外敷;或以生白附子或鲜蟾蜍皮外敷,或用大黄粉以醋调敷。

1.2.3　乳房肿瘤

包括乳房良性肿瘤和恶性肿瘤,这里简述乳核与乳岩。

1.2.3.1　乳核

乳核是发生在乳房部最常见的良性肿瘤。相当于西医的乳腺纤维腺瘤。

【诊断】

多发于青年女性,乳房内圆形或椭圆形肿块,直径大多在 0.5～5cm 之间,边界清楚,质地坚实,表面光滑,按之有硬橡皮球之弹性,活动度大,触诊常有滑脱感。一般生长缓慢,妊娠期可迅速增大,应排除恶变可能。

B 超检查,钼钯 X 线摄片可协助诊断。

【治疗】

内治　肝气郁结证,以逍遥散加减;血瘀痰凝证,以逍遥散合桃红四物汤加减,月经不调兼以调摄冲任。

外治　阳和解凝膏掺黑退消外贴,7 天换药 1 次。

其他疗法:一般应作手术切除,做病理检查。

1.2.3.2　乳岩

乳岩是指乳房部的恶性肿瘤。相当于西医的乳腺癌。

【诊断】

发病年龄一般在 40～60 岁,绝经期妇女发病率相对较高。乳癌可分为一般类型乳腺癌及特殊类型乳腺癌。

一般类型乳腺癌:常为乳房内无痛肿块,边界不清,质地坚硬,表面不光滑,不易推动,常与皮肤粘连,出现病灶中心酒窝征,个别可伴乳头溢液。后期随着癌肿逐渐增大,产生不同程度疼痛,皮肤可呈橘皮样水肿、变色;乳头内缩或抬高,偶可见到皮肤溃疡。癌肿转移至腋下及锁骨上时,可触及肿大淋巴结。

特殊类型乳腺癌:包括炎性癌、湿疹样癌等。

钼靶 X 线摄片,B 超检查可帮助诊断。病理切片检查有助于确诊。

【治疗】

早期诊断是乳岩治疗的关键。原则上以手术治疗为主。中医药治疗多用于晚期患者,特别对手术后患者有良好的调治作用,对放、化疗有减毒增效作用,可提高病人生存质量,延长生存期。

内治　肝郁痰凝证,以神效瓜蒌散合开郁散加减;冲任失调证,以二仙汤合开郁散加减;正虚毒炽证,以八珍汤加减;气血两亏证,以人参养荣汤加味;脾虚胃弱证以参苓白术散或理中汤加减。除以上几种常见类型外,放、化疗后胃阴虚,口腔糜烂,牙龈出血等,治宜清养胃阴,方用益胃汤加减。

外治　适用于有手术禁忌证,或已远处广泛转移,已不适宜手术者。初起用阿魏消痞膏外贴;溃后用海浮散或冰狮散、红油膏外敷;坏死组织脱落后,改用生肌玉红膏、生肌散外敷。

其他疗法　手术治疗、化疗、放疗、内分泌治疗;中成药:可选用犀黄丸、醒消丸、小金丹治疗。

1.3　瘿

瘿是甲状腺疾病的总称。其特点是:发于甲状腺部,或为漫肿,或为结块,或有灼痛,多数皮色不变,可随吞咽动作上下移动,或伴有烦热、心悸、多汗及月经不调,甚至闭经等症状。包括西医学的单纯性甲状腺肿、甲状腺腺瘤、甲状腺囊肿、甲状腺癌、甲状腺炎及甲状腺机能亢进等。

1.3.1 肉瘿

肉瘿是瘿病中较常见的一种,其临床特点是颈前喉结一侧或两侧结块,柔韧而圆,如肉之团,随吞咽动作而上下移动,发展缓慢。好发于青年女性及中年人。相当于西医的甲状腺腺瘤或囊肿。

【诊断】

结喉正中一侧或双侧有单个肿块,呈半圆形,表面光滑,可随吞咽动作上下移动,按之不痛,生长缓慢,一般无明显全身症状。部分患者可伴甲状腺功能亢进征象,少数患者可发生癌变。

超声波探测,同位素 B1 碘扫描可帮助诊断。

【治疗】

内治 气滞痰凝证,逍遥散合海藻玉壶汤加减;气阴两虚证,生脉散合海藻玉壶汤加减。

外治 阳和解凝膏掺黑退消或桂麝散外敷。

其他疗法 针刺、手术治疗。

1.3.2 石瘿

瘿病坚硬如石不可移动者,称为石瘿。相当于西医的甲状腺癌。

【诊断】

颈前肿块，质地坚硬如石，表面凹凸不平，推之不移，并可出现吞咽时移动受限。可伴有疼痛，若颈丛神经浅支受侵，则耳、枕、肩部剧痛。若肿块压迫，引起喉头移位或侵犯喉部神经时，可引起呼吸或吞咽困难。有时颈部出现淋巴结肿大。

可以采用甲状腺同位素 B1 碘扫描、B 型超声、CT 检查及病理学检查以明确诊断。

【治疗】

内治　痰瘀内结证，以海藻玉壶汤合桃红四物汤治疗；瘀热伤阴证，以通窍活血汤合养阴清肺汤加减。

外治　阳和解凝膏掺阿魏粉敷贴；肿块疼痛灼热者，可用生商陆根捣烂外敷。

其他疗法　石瘿一旦确诊后，宜早期手术切除，或局部放射治疗。

1.4　瘤岩

瘤是瘀血、痰滞、浊气停留于机体组织间而产生的结块。相当于西医的部分体表良性肿瘤。

岩是发生于体表的恶性肿物的统称，为外科疾病中最凶险者。因其质地坚硬，表面凹凸不平，形如岩石而得名。相当于西医的体表恶性肿瘤。

这里瘤、岩合述，并专论血瘤、肉瘤、茧唇、失荣、肾岩翻花五种瘤、岩代表性疾病。

1.4.1　血瘤

血瘤是指体表血络扩张,纵横丛集而形成的肿瘤。相当于西医的血管瘤。常见的有毛细血管瘤和海绵状血管瘤。

【诊断】

毛细血管瘤,多发于儿童颜面、颈部,多数表现为在皮肤上有红色丘疹或小的红斑,逐渐长大,界限清楚,大小不等,质软可压缩,色泽为鲜红色或紫红色,压之可褪色,抬手复原。

海绵状血管瘤,表现为质地柔软似海绵,常呈局限性半球形、扁平或高出皮面的隆起物,肿物有很大压缩性,可因体位下垂而充盈,或随患肢抬高而缩小,在瘤内有时可扪及颗粒状的静脉石硬结,外伤后可引起出血,继发感染,可形成慢性出血性溃疡。

【治疗】

内治　心肾火毒证,以芩连二母丸合凉血地黄汤加减;肝经火旺证,以丹栀逍遥散合清肝芦荟丸加减;脾统失司证,以顺气归脾丸加减。

外治　对小面积毛细血管瘤及海绵状血管瘤可用五妙水仙膏外搽;清凉膏合藤黄膏外敷,包扎固定;若肿瘤出血,可用云南白药掺敷伤口。

其他疗法　注射疗法,消痔灵注射液加 1% 普鲁卡因,按 1 ：1 混合,注射硬化;另外还有手术疗法、冷冻疗法、放射疗法。

1.4.2　茧唇

茧唇是发生于唇部的岩肿,因其外形似蚕茧而得名。相当于西医的唇癌。

【诊断】

本病发病缓慢,多见于老年男性,病变多发于下唇的中、外 1/3 交界处的红缘部,口角及上唇者较少见。多在良性病变的基础上发生,如长期不愈的角化增生、白斑、破裂或乳头状瘤等。初起为局限性硬结,状如豆粒,渐渐增大,开始多无疼痛,进而溃破如翻花,时流血水并伴疼痛,张口进食困难。病情进一步发展,患者颌下及颈下淋巴结可肿大固定,常为癌肿转移之征象。

【治疗】

内治　心脾火炽证,以清凉甘露饮加减;脾胃实热证,以凉隔散合清胃散加减;阴虚火旺证,以知柏地黄汤加减。

外治　皮癌净外敷,每日或隔日 1 次;蟾酥丸加醋研磨后外敷患部。

其他疗法　中成药以犀黄丸、小金片内服;西医可采用手术、放疗、化疗、激光治疗。

1.4.3　失荣

失荣是发于颈部及耳之前后的岩肿,因其晚期气血亏乏,面容憔悴,形体消瘦,状如树木枝叶发枯,失去荣华而命名。相当于西医的颈部淋巴结转移癌和原发性恶性肿瘤。

【诊断】

一般表现为颈部淋巴结肿大,生长较快,质地坚硬。病变开始时多为单发结节,可活动;后期肿块体积增大,数量增多,融合成团块或联结成串,表面不平,固定不移。日久癌肿溃破,疮面渗流血水,高低不平,形似翻花状。其肿痛可向面部、胸部、肩背部扩展。

进行全面细致的体格检查,寻找原发病灶或作活组织病理检查以协助确诊。

【治疗】

内治 初期为肝郁痰凝,痰瘀互结,以开郁散治疗;中期,毒聚正衰,以和营散坚丸加减;后期,气血衰败,以香贝养荣汤治疗。

外治 初期,以阿魏化痞膏外贴;溃后,用生肌玉红膏掺海乳散外敷。

其他疗法 中成药,以犀黄丸内服;局部病变放射治疗或配合全身化疗、手术治疗等。

1.4.4 肾岩

阴茎属肾,岩肿生于阴茎,故名"肾岩",相当于西医的阴茎癌。

【诊断】

本病多发于中老年人。初起时在包皮系带附近、阴茎头部、冠状沟部或尿道口处,可见丘疹、红斑、结节、疣状增生等,逐渐增大、刺痒,甚至破溃,严重者阴茎溃烂脱落。局部可见淋巴结转移。本病早期一般无明显全身症状,晚期可出现发热、消瘦、贫血等。

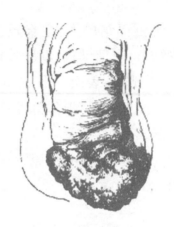

图 5　肾岩

行病理切片检查可以明确诊断。

【治疗】

内治　湿浊瘀结证,以三妙丸合散肿溃坚汤加减;火毒炽盛证,以龙胆泻肝汤合四妙勇安汤加减;阴虚火旺证,以知柏地黄丸合大补阴丸加减。

外治法　① 岩肿溃烂不洁,用五五丹或千金散撒于疮面,或用红灵丹油膏外敷,腐蚀至癌肿平复后,改用九一丹。如创面渗血可掺海浮散,外敷生肌玉红膏。创面清洁后,改用红油膏或白玉膏。② 皮癌净外敷,1 日 1 次或隔日 1 次。③氟脲嘧啶软膏,外搽患部,1 日 2 次。

其他疗法　化疗,放疗,手术行阴茎局部切除、阴茎部分切除或阴茎全切除术。

1.5　肛门直肠疾病

肛门直肠疾病是指发生于肛门直肠部位的疾病。常见的有痔、肛隐窝炎、肛裂、肛痈、肛漏、脱肛、息肉痔、锁肛痔等，在古代文献中统称为痔疮、痔瘘。

1.5.1 痔

痔是直肠下段黏膜下和肛管皮肤下的静脉丛淤血、扩张和屈曲所形成的静脉团，是最常见的肛肠疾病。

【诊断】

主要表现为无痛性便后出鲜血，痔块脱出，肛周潮湿、瘙痒，坠胀疼痛等。

内痔，由直肠上静脉丛形成，位于齿状线以上，表面为直肠黏膜所覆盖，根据内痔脱出情况可分为三期。

外痔，由直肠下静脉丛形成，位于齿状线以下，表面为肛管皮肤覆盖。主要有血栓性外痔、静脉曲张性外痔、结缔组织外痔和炎性外痔。

混合痔，由直肠上、下静脉丛均发生曲张，称为混合痔，表面为直肠黏膜和肛管皮肤所覆盖，痔块逐渐发展，脱出肛门外可形成环形痔或嵌顿性痔。

【治疗】

内治 多适用于Ⅰ、Ⅱ期内痔，或嵌顿痔有继发感染，或年老体弱，或内痔兼有其他严重慢性疾病，不宜手术治疗者。风热肠燥证，以凉血地黄汤加减，大便秘结者，加润肠汤；湿热下注证，以脏连丸加减；气滞血瘀证，以止痛如神汤加减；脾虚气陷证，以补中益气汤加减，血虚者合四物汤。

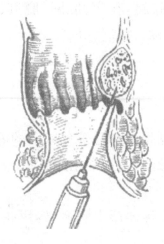

图 6　内痔注射疗法

外治　适用于各期内痔及内痔嵌顿肿痛等。熏洗法,常用五倍子汤、苦参汤等先熏后洗,或湿热敷;外敷法,将药物敷于患处,用消痔膏、五倍子散;塞药法,将药物制成栓剂,塞如痔疮栓。

其他疗法　插药疗法,该疗法是中医学治疗内痔的一种有效方法。它是将药末与糯米粉混合后加水制成两头尖、形如钉子的药条,插入痔核内,使痔核产生无菌性炎症反应,纤维组织增生或干枯坏死,从而使痔核萎缩或脱落,达到治疗目的;注射法,根据其药理作用的不同,分为硬化萎缩和坏死枯脱两种方法;结扎疗法,目前常用的有贯穿结扎法和胶圈套扎法两种;手术疗法,包括痔单纯切除术、痔环形切除术、血栓性外痔剥离术等。

1.5.2　肛痈

肛痈是指肛管直肠周围间隙发生急慢性感染而形成的

脓肿。相当于现代医学的肛门直肠周围脓肿。

【诊断】

发病男性多于女性,尤以青壮年为多,主要表现为肛门周围疼痛、肿胀、有结块,伴有不同程度发热、倦怠等全身症状。

由于脓肿的部位和深浅不同,症状也有差异,如提肛肌以上的间隙脓肿,位置深隐,全身症状重,而局部症状轻;提肛肌以下的间隙脓肿,部位浅,局部红、肿、热、痛明显,而全身症状较轻。

【治疗】

肛痈的治疗以手术治疗为主,注意预防肛漏的形成。

内治　热毒蕴结证,以仙方活命饮、黄连解毒汤加减;火毒炽盛证以透脓散加减;阴虚毒恋证以青蒿鳖甲汤合三妙丸加减。

外治　初起,实证用金黄膏、黄连膏外敷,位置深隐者,可用金黄散调糊灌肠;虚证用冲和膏或阳和解凝膏外敷;成脓,宜早期切开引流,并根据脓肿部位深浅和病情缓急选择手术方法;溃后,用九一丹纱条引流,脓尽改用生肌散纱条,日久成瘘者,按肛漏处理。

其他疗法　手术方法包括脓肿一次切开法、一次切开挂线法、分次手术疗法。

1.5.3　肛漏

肛漏是指直肠或肛管与周围皮肤相通所形成的瘘管。

【诊断】

瘘外口流出少量脓性、血性、黏液性分泌物。由于有分泌物刺激,肛门部潮湿、瘙痒,有时有湿疹形成。肛门视诊可见外口,以探针探查,常可找到内口。

可分为低位单纯性肛漏、低位复杂性肛漏、高位单纯性肛漏、高位复杂性肛漏四种类型。

X线碘油造影术可显示瘘管走行、深浅、有无分支及内口的位置,与直肠及周围脏器的关系等,为手术提供可靠的依据。

【治疗】

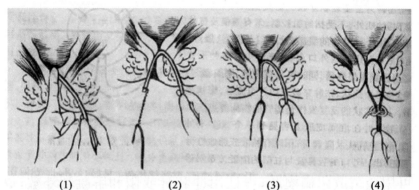

(1) 手指协助控针由外口探入内口;(2) 弯曲探针前端,将其拉到肛外;(3) 探针前端缚一丝线,并接上一橡皮筋;(4) 退出控针,将橡皮筋由瘘管拉出,用丝线结扎.

图 7　肛瘘挂线疗法

内治　湿热下注证以二妙丸合萆薢渗湿汤加减;正虚邪恋证,托里消毒饮加减;阴液亏损证,以青蒿鳖甲汤加减。

其他疗法　以手术治疗为主。将瘘管全部切开,必要时可将瘘管周围的瘢痕组织作适当修剪,使之引流通畅,创口逐渐愈合。手术成败的关键,在于正确地找到内口,并将内口切开或切除,否则创口就不能愈合,即使暂时愈合,日久又会复发。目前常用的手术疗法,有挂线疗法、切开疗法、切开与挂线相结合疗法等三种。

1.5.4 肛裂

肛管的皮肤全层纵行裂开并形成感染性溃疡者称肛裂。

【诊断】

临床上以肛门周期性疼痛、出血、便秘为主要特点。

早期肛裂,仅在肛管皮肤见一个小的溃疡,创面浅而色鲜红,边缘整齐而有弹性;陈旧性肛裂,底深而不整齐,质硬,边缘增厚纤维化,肉芽灰白。裂口上端的肛门瓣和肛乳头水肿,形成肛乳头肥大;下端皮肤因炎症、水肿及静脉、淋巴回流障碍,形成袋装皮赘向下突出于肛门外,称为前哨痔。

【治疗】

早期肛裂可采用保守治疗,陈旧性肛裂多需采用手术治疗。

内治 血热肠燥证,治以凉血地黄汤合脾约麻仁丸;阴虚津亏证,以润肠汤治疗;气滞血瘀证,以六磨汤加红花、桃仁、赤芍等。

外治 早期肛裂,可用生肌玉红膏蘸生肌散外涂;1∶5000 高锰酸钾、苦参汤或花椒食盐水液坐浴;陈旧性肛裂,可用七三丹或枯痔散等腐蚀药搽于裂口,二三天腐脱后,改用生肌白玉膏、生肌散收口。或用长强穴封闭疗法。

其他疗法 陈旧性肛裂和非手术疗法治疗无效的早期肛裂,可考虑扩肛法、切开疗法、肛裂侧切术、纵切横缝法等。

1.6   泌尿男性疾病

泌尿男性疾病包括泌尿系统和男性生殖系统疾病。

1.6.1   男性不育

男性不育是指育龄夫妇同居 2 年以上，性生活正常，未采取任何避孕措施，女方有受孕能力，由丁男方原因而致女方不能怀孕的一类疾病。

【诊断】

对不育症的诊断，应从以下几方面进行。

了解病史，根据患者的职业、既往史、个人生活史、婚姻史来寻找病因。进行体格检查，了解发育营养状况，有无精索静脉曲张等。实验室检查，包括精液检查、睾丸活组织检查、生殖内分泌测定、遗传学检查等。

【治疗】

内治　肾阳虚衰证，金匮肾气丸合五子衍宗丸或羊睾丸汤加减；肾阴不足证，左归丸合五子衍宗丸加减，若阴虚火旺者，宜滋阴降火，用知柏地黄汤加减；肝郁气滞证，柴胡疏肝散合五子衍宗丸加减；湿热下注证，程氏萆薢分清饮加减；气血两虚证，十全大补汤加减。

1.6.2   慢性前列腺炎

慢性前列腺炎是中青年男性常见的一种生殖系统综合征。

临床上有急性和慢性、有菌性和无菌性、特异性和非特异性的区别,其中以慢性无菌性非特异性前列腺炎最为多见。

【诊断】

临床症状表现不一,患者可出现轻微的尿频、尿急、尿痛、尿道内灼热不适或排尿不净之感;有的在排尿终末或大便用力时,自尿道滴出少量乳白色的前列腺液。多数患者可伴会阴部坠胀隐痛。部分患者因病程较长可出现阳痿、早泄、遗精或射精痛等,或头晕、耳鸣、失眠多梦、腰酸乏力等神经衰弱症状。

直肠指检,前列腺多为正常大小,或稍大或稍小,触诊可有轻度压痛。有的前列腺可表现为软硬不均或缩小变硬等异常现象。

前列腺分泌物涂片检查有助于诊断。

【治疗】

主张综合治疗,注意调护。临床以辨证论治为主,抓住肾虚(本)、湿热(标)、瘀滞(变)三个基本病理环节,分清主次,权衡用药。

内治 湿热蕴结证,八正散或龙胆泻肝汤加减;气滞血瘀证,前列腺汤加减;阴虚火旺证,知柏地黄汤加减;肾阳虚损证,济生肾气丸加减。

外治 葱归溻肿汤坐浴,每次 20 分钟,每日 2 次;野菊花栓或前列栓塞肛门内约 3~4cm,每日 2 次。

其他疗法 针对病原体,根据药敏试验合理选用抗生素;理疗、局部超短波透热或局部有效抗生素离子透入治疗。

1.6.3 前列腺增生症

前列腺增生症俗称前列腺肥大,是老年男性的常见疾病之一。

【诊断】

本病多见于 55 岁以上的老年男性患者。逐渐出现进行性尿频,以夜间为明显,并伴排尿困难,尿线变细。部分患者由于尿液长期不能排尽,致膀胱残余尿增多,而出现假性尿失禁。在发病过程中,常因受寒、劳累、憋尿、便秘等,而发生急性尿潴留。严重者可引起肾功能损伤,而出现肾功能不全的一系列症状。有些患者可并发尿路感染、膀胱结石、疝气或脱肛等。

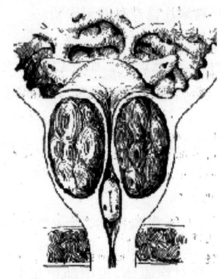

图 8　前列腺增生

直肠指检,前列腺常有不同程度的增大,表面光滑,中等硬度而富有弹性,中央沟变浅或消失。B 型超声、CT、膀胱尿道造影、膀胱镜及尿流动力学等检查可协助诊断。

【治疗】

治疗应以通为用,温肾益气、活血利尿是其基本的治疗法则。出现并发症时应采用中西医综合疗法。

内治　湿热下注证,八正散加减;脾肾气虚证,补中益气汤加菟丝子、肉苁蓉、补骨脂、车前子等;气滞血瘀证,沉香散加减;肾阴亏虚证,知柏地黄丸加丹参、琥珀、王不留行、地龙等;肾阳不足证,济生肾气丸加减。

外治　可以采用中药外敷、灌肠治疗,必要时可行导尿术。

其他可配合手术疗法、西药治疗、物理疗法、针灸疗法。

1.7　周围血管病

周围血管疾病是指发生于心、脑血管以外的血管疾病。可分为动脉病和静脉病。动脉病包括血栓闭塞性脉管炎、动脉硬化性闭塞症、动脉栓塞、多发性大动脉炎、动脉瘤等。另外,还包括肢端动脉舒缩功能紊乱疾病,如雷诺病(症)、红斑性肢痛症等。静脉病包括血栓性浅静脉炎、深静脉血栓形成、深静脉瓣膜功能不全、静脉曲张等。

中医称周围血管为经脉、脉管,故将周围血管疾病统称为"脉管病"。

1.7.1　臁疮

臁疮是指发生于小腿臁骨部位的慢性皮肤溃疡。常为筋瘤的后期并发症,相当于西医的慢性下肢溃疡。

【诊断】

本病多见于久立、久行者,常为筋瘤病的后期并发症之一。

初起小腿肿胀,有沉重感,局部青筋怒胀,渐渐出现浅静脉炎、色素沉着、淤积性皮炎、湿疹等一系列静脉功能不全表现,继而在小腿下 1/3 处内臁或外臁持续漫肿、苔癣样变的皮肤出现裂缝,糜烂、滋水淋漓,溃疡形成,后期疮口下陷,边缘高起形如缸口,疮面肉色灰白或秽暗,滋水秽浊,疮面周围皮色暗红或紫黑,或四周起湿疹而痒,日久不愈。继发感染则溃疡化脓,或并发出血。严重时溃疡可扩大上至膝下到足背,深达骨膜。少数病人可因缠绵多年不愈,蕴毒深沉而导致癌变。

下肢静脉瓣膜功能试验有助于判断瓣膜功能。下肢静脉血管造影、超声多普勒血流检测等方法检查可协助诊断。

【治疗】

内治 湿热下注证,二妙丸合五神汤加减;气虚血瘀证,补阳还五汤合四妙汤加减。

外治 初期,局部红肿,溃破渗液较多者,宜用中药煎汤外洗。局部红肿,渗液量少者,宜金黄膏薄敷。后期,用七层丹麻油调,摊贴疮面,并用绷带缠缚。腐肉已脱,露新肉者,用生肌散外盖生肌玉红膏。周围有湿疹者,用青黛散调麻油盖贴。

其他疗法 西医治疗小腿溃疡主要采取手术、局部治疗、穿医用弹力袜等。

1.7.2 脱疽

脱疽是指发于四肢末端,严重时趾(指)节坏疽脱落的一种慢性周围血管疾病,又称脱骨疽。相当于西医学的血栓闭塞性脉管炎、动脉硬化性闭塞症和糖尿病足。

【诊断】

血栓闭塞性脉管炎多发于青年男性,下肢多见,患者多有受冷、潮湿、嗜烟、外伤等病史。动脉硬化性闭塞症多发于老年人,常伴有高脂血症、高血压和动脉硬化病史,常累及大、中动脉。糖尿病足多伴有糖尿病病史,可累及大动脉和微小动脉。

根据疾病的发展过程,临床一般可分为三期:局部缺血期、营养障碍期、坏死期或坏疽期。

肢体超声多普勒、血流图、甲皱微循环、动脉造影及血脂、血糖等检查,有助于鉴别诊断,了解病情严重程度。

【治疗】

本病轻症可单用中、西药治疗,重症应中西医结合治疗。中医以辨证论治为主,但活血化瘀法贯穿始终,常配合静脉滴注活血化瘀药物,以建立侧支循环,改善肢体血运。

内治 寒湿阻络证,阳和汤加减;血脉瘀阻证,桃红四物汤加减;湿热毒盛证,四妙勇安汤加减;热毒伤阴证,顾步汤加减;气阴两虚证,黄芪鳖甲煎加减。各型可配合毛冬青煎水内服;丹参注射液静脉滴注。病因治疗:动脉硬化性闭塞症,应用降血脂、降血压药物;糖尿病足,积极控制血糖,规范治疗,防治感染,促进肢体血液循环的恢复。

外治 未溃期,选用冲和膏、红灵丹油膏外敷;已溃,溃疡面积较小者,外敷生肌玉红膏;溃疡面积较大,坏死组织难以脱落者,可先用冰片锌氧油软化创面硬结痂皮,按疏松程度,依次清除坏死痂皮,先除软组织,后除腐骨,彻底的清创术必须待炎症完全消退后方可施行,或实行截肢术。

1.8　其他外科疾病

其他外科疾病包括冻疮、烧伤、虫兽咬伤、破伤风和肠痈等。这里介绍烧伤。

烧伤

烧伤是由于热力（火焰、灼热的气体、液体或固体）、电能、化学物质、放射线等作用于人体而引起的一种局部或全身急性损伤性疾病。

【诊断】

烧伤深度一般采用三度四分法，即Ⅰ度、Ⅱ度（又分浅Ⅱ度、深Ⅱ度）和Ⅲ度烧伤。

为了设计治疗方案，需要对烧伤的严重程度进行分类，一般分为4类：轻度烧伤、中度烧伤、重度烧伤、特重烧伤。

【治疗】

内治　火毒伤津证，黄连解毒汤、银花甘草汤、犀角地黄汤或清营汤加减；阴伤阳脱证，四逆汤、参附汤合生脉散加味；火毒内陷证，清营汤或黄连解毒汤合犀角地黄汤加减，神昏谵语者，加服安宫牛黄丸或紫雪丹；气血两虚证，托里消毒散或八珍汤加金银花、黄芪；脾虚阴伤证，益胃汤合参苓白术散加减。

外治

①在防治休克的基础上，局部清创。

②初期，小面积Ⅰ、Ⅱ度烧伤可外涂京万红烫伤药膏、清凉膏、紫草膏、万花油等，暴露或包扎；或用地榆粉、大黄粉各等份，麻油调敷后包扎，隔日换药一次。

较大面积的Ⅱ度烧伤，皮肤无破损者，抽出疱内液体后，用虎地酊喷洒创面,每日数次;水疱完整或水疱已破者,剪去破损外皮,外用湿润烧伤膏。

Ⅲ度烧伤可外涂碘伏,保持焦痂干燥,防止感染。全身情况好者,于3～6天后采取分批多次切痂并植皮,或保痂开窗植皮;亦可外用水火烫伤膏、创灼膏等脱痂。

③中期,创面感染者,可根据创面大小、感染性质,采用不同的外用药和方法。一般小面积感染创面可外用黄连膏、红油膏、生肌玉红膏外敷;较大面积感染创面,渗液较多,可选用2‰黄连液、2‰黄柏液、10‰虎杖液湿敷;痂下积脓者,要尽快去痂引流,用上述药液浸泡或湿敷。或者根据脓液细菌培养及药敏试验用药。

④后期,腐脱新生时,用生肌白玉膏、生肌玉红膏或生肌散外敷。

其他疗法 包括现场急救和西医治疗。

1.9 皮肤及性传播疾病

发生于人体皮肤、黏膜及皮肤附属器的疾病统称为皮肤病。性传播疾病是指通过性接触、类似性行为及间接接触所感染的一组传染性疾病,简称为"性病"。

1.9.1 癣

癣是发生在表皮、毛发、指(趾)甲的浅部真菌皮肤病。这里只讨论浅在的常见皮肤真菌病,如头癣、手脚癣、体癣等。

【诊断】

(1)临床表现

①白秃疮,相当于西医的白癣。青春期可自愈,秃发也能再生,不遗留瘢痕。

②肥疮,相当于西医的黄癣。病变日久毛囊被破坏而成永久性脱发。

③鹅掌风,相当于西医的手癣。皮疹特点初起为掌心或指缝水疱或掌部皮肤角化脱屑、水疱。若反复发作后,致手掌皮肤肥厚,枯槁干裂,疼痛,屈伸不利,损害若侵及指甲而成甲癣。

④脚湿气,相当于西医的脚癣。分为水疱型、糜烂型、脱屑型,但常以一二种皮肤损害为主。

⑤圆癣,相当于西医的体癣。圆癣的皮损特征为环形、多环形,边界清楚,中心消退,外围扩张的斑块。自觉瘙痒,搔抓日久,皮肤可呈苔藓样变。

⑥紫白癜风,相当于西医的花斑癣,淡褐,灰褐至深褐色皮损,或轻度色素减退,或附少许糠秕状细鳞屑,常常反复发作。

(2)实验室检查 真菌直接镜检、真菌培养进行菌种鉴定。深部真菌病需做病变组织的病理学检查。

【治疗】

本病以杀虫止痒为主要治法,必须彻底治疗。抗真菌西药有一定优势,可中西药合用。癣病以外治为主,若皮损广泛,自觉症状较重,或抓破染毒者,则宜内治、外治相结合为宜。

内治 风湿毒聚证,消风散加减;湿热下注证,湿重于热者,用萆薢渗湿汤,湿热兼瘀者,用五神汤,湿热并重者,用龙胆泻肝汤。

外治 各种癣可根据不同情况选用 1 号癣药水、2 号癣药水、3％硼酸溶液、二矾汤,或半边莲 60g 煎汤待温,浸泡 15 分钟,皮脂膏或雄黄膏等外搽。

其他疗法 西医治疗,内服抗真菌药物如灰黄霉素、伊曲康唑、特比萘芬等。外用可选 5％～10％硫黄软膏、50％丙二醇、咪唑类及丙烯胺类霜剂或溶液。

1.9.2 湿疮

湿疮是一种过敏性炎症性皮肤病。相当于西医的湿疹。

【诊断】

(1)急性湿疮 相当于西医急性湿疹。本病起病较快,皮损常为对称性,原发性和多形性(常有红斑、潮红、丘疹、丘疱疹、水疱、脓疱、流滋、结痂并存)。可发于身体的任何部位,亦可泛发全身,但常在头面、耳后、手足、会阴部位对称分布。

(2)亚急性湿疮 相当于西医亚急性湿疹。常由急性湿疮未能及时治疗,或处理失当,致病程迁延所致。亦可初发即呈亚急性湿疮。皮损较急性湿疮轻,以丘疹、结痂、鳞屑为主,仅有少量水疱及轻度糜烂。自觉剧烈瘙痒,夜间尤甚。

(3)慢性湿疮 相当于西医慢性湿疹。皮损多局限于某一部位,表现为皮肤肥厚粗糙,触之较硬,色暗红或紫褐色,皮纹显著或呈苔藓样变。部分皮损可出现新的丘疹或水疱。患者自觉瘙痒,呈阵发性,夜间或精神紧张,饮酒、食辛辣发物时瘙痒加剧。病程较长,反复发作,时轻时重。

【治疗】

本病以清热利湿止痒为主要治法。急性者,以清热利湿为主;慢性者以养血润肤为主。外治宜用温和的药物,以免加重病情。

内治　湿热蕴肤证,龙胆泻肝汤合萆薢渗湿汤加减;湿热浸淫证,龙胆泻肝汤合五味消毒饮加减;脾虚湿蕴证,除湿胃苓汤或参苓白术散加减;血虚风燥证,当归饮子或四物消风饮加减。

外治

①急性湿疮:初起可选用中药苦参、黄柏、地肤子、荆芥等煎汤温洗;若水疱糜烂、渗出明显时,可选用黄柏、生地榆、马齿苋、野菊花等煎汤湿敷,再用青黛散麻油调搽;急性湿疮后期滋水减少时,可选黄连软膏、青黛膏外搽。

②亚急性湿疮:外治原则为消炎、止痒、干燥、收敛,选用三黄洗剂、3%黑豆馏油、10%生地榆氧化锌油外搽。

③慢性湿疮:一般可外搽青黛膏、5%硫黄软膏、5%~10%复方松馏油软膏。

其他疗法　西医疗法,选用抗组胺药、镇静剂、维生素类药物。外用药,氧化锌油、3%硼酸溶液湿敷,亦可用糖皮质激素霜剂外搽。

1.9.3　牛皮癣

牛皮癣是一种皮肤状如牛领之皮,厚而且坚的慢性瘙痒性皮肤病。相当于西医的神经性皮炎。

【诊断】

发病部位大多数见于颈项部、额部,其次为尾骶、肘窝、腘窝,亦可见腰背、两髋、外阴、肛周、腹股沟及四肢等处。常呈对称性分布,亦可沿皮肤皱折或皮神经分布呈线状排列。

皮损初起有聚集倾向的扁平丘疹,干燥而结实,皮色正常或淡褐色,表面光泽。久之融合成片,逐渐扩大,皮肤增厚干燥成席纹状,稍有脱屑。长期搔抓,皮肤浸润肥厚,嵴沟明显,呈苔藓化。自觉阵发性奇痒,入夜尤甚;搔之不知痛楚。情绪波动时,瘙痒随之加剧。

局限型:皮损仅见于颈项等局部,为少数境界清楚的苔藓样肥厚斑片。

泛发型:分布较广泛,以肘窝、腘窝、四肢、面部及躯干为多,甚至泛发全身各处,皮损同局限型。

本病慢性病程,常多年不愈,易反复发作。

【治疗】

本病治疗以疏风清热、养血润燥为治则。对继发感染,应采用抗菌药物,及时控制感染。

内治　肝经化火证,龙胆泻肝汤加减;风湿蕴肤证,消风散加减;血虚风燥证,当归饮子加减。

外治　肝经化火,风湿蕴肤,用三黄洗剂外搽;血虚风燥,外用油膏加热烘疗法;羊蹄根散,醋调搽患处,每天 1～2 次。

其他疗法　包括针刺疗法、梅花针疗法、穴位注射疗法。

1.9.4　白疕

白疕因其"肤如疹疥,色白而痒,搔起白皮"而得名,是一种常见的易于复发的炎症性皮肤病。相当于西医的银屑病。

【诊断】

（1）临床表现　本病好发于青壮年，男性多于女性，有一定遗传倾向；大多数冬季发病或加重，夏季减轻，数年后与季节变化关系不明显。

根据白疕的临床特征，可分为寻常型、脓疱型、关节型、红皮病型四种类型。

（2）实验室和其他辅助检查　常见血白细胞增高及血沉加快；脓疱型细菌培养阴性；组织病理学检查可见不同表现。

【治疗】

寻常型以中医辨证论治为主要治疗方法；脓疱型、关节型、红皮病型应以中西医结合治疗。

内治　血热内蕴证，犀角地黄汤加减；血虚风燥证，当归饮子加减；气血瘀滞证，桃红四物汤加减；湿毒蕴阻证，萆薢渗湿汤加减；火毒炽盛证，清瘟败毒饮加减。

外治　进行期皮损宜用温和之剂，可用黄连膏、普连膏；静止期、退行期皮损可用药渣煎水，放温，洗浴浸泡患处，再外涂黄连膏。

其他疗法　西医治疗，常选用抗生素、维生素类、免疫抑制剂、免疫疗法、静脉封闭疗法及物理疗法；针刺、耳针、刺络拔罐疗法有一定效果。

1.9.5　红蝴蝶疮

红蝴蝶疮是一种可累及皮肤和全身多脏器的自身免疫性疾病。相当于西医的红斑狼疮。

【诊断】

（1）临床表现　本病分为盘状红蝴蝶疮与系统性红蝴蝶疮，以后者多见。

①盘状红蝴蝶疮：多见于 20～40 岁左右的女性，皮损好发于面部，亦可发于手背、指侧、唇红部、肩胛部等处。

②系统性红蝴蝶疮：多见于青年及中年女性，男女之比约为 1 ：10。

本病早期表现多种多样，症状多不明显，皮肤、黏膜损害表现多样，初起可单个器官受累，或多个系统同时被侵犯。可有发热，关节、肌肉疼痛，肾脏损害，心血管系统病变，呼吸系统病变，神经系统病变，淋巴系统、造血系统及眼底病变。

（2）实验室检查　全血细胞分析、尿液分析、免疫学检查有助于诊断。

【治疗】

中医治疗多从补益肝肾、活血化瘀、祛风解毒入手。本病病情复杂，临床多采用中西医结合治疗。

内治　热毒炽盛证，犀角地黄汤合黄连解毒汤加减；阴虚火旺证，六味地黄丸合大补阴丸、清骨散加减；脾肾阳虚证，附桂八味丸合真武汤加减；脾虚肝旺证，四君子汤合丹栀逍遥散加减；气滞血瘀证，逍遥散合血府逐瘀汤加减。

外治　皮损处涂白玉膏或黄柏霜，每天 1～2 次。

其他疗法　西医治疗，对急性发作或重型病例，宜选用皮质类固醇激素、免疫抑制剂等治疗；中成药，昆明山海棠片、雷公藤多苷片、青蒿浸膏片、复方金荞片等药物口服治疗。

1.9.6　梅毒

梅毒是由梅毒螺旋体所引起的一种全身性、慢性性传播疾病。属于中医"霉疮"、"疳疮"、"花柳病"等范畴。

【诊断】

(1)临床表现　一般有不洁性交史,或性伴侣有梅毒病史。

①一期梅毒,主要表现为疳疮(硬下疳),局部淋巴肿大;二期梅毒,主要表现为杨梅疮,出现皮肤黏膜损害、骨损害、眼梅毒、神经梅毒等;三期梅毒,亦称晚期梅毒,主要表现为杨梅结毒。除皮肤黏膜损害外,常侵犯多个脏器。

②潜伏梅毒(隐性梅毒),无临床症状,血清反应阳性,排除其他可引起血清反应阳性的疾病存在,脑脊液正常,这类病称为潜伏梅毒。

③胎传梅毒(先天梅毒),胎传梅毒是母体内的梅毒螺旋体由血液通过胎盘传入到胎儿血液中,导致胎儿感染的梅毒。胎传梅毒常有严重的内脏损害,对患儿的健康影响很大,病死率高。

(2)实验室检查　梅毒螺旋体抗原血清试验阳性、聚合酯链反应检查梅毒螺旋体核糖核酸阳性或组织、分泌物查到梅毒螺旋体可确诊。

【治疗】

梅毒的治疗,首选青霉素类药物、四环素或红霉素等药物治疗,而中医药治疗梅毒,一般仅作为驱梅治疗中的辅助疗法。

内治　肝经湿热证,龙胆泻肝汤酌加土茯苓、虎杖;血热蕴毒证,清营汤合桃红四物汤加减;毒结筋骨证,五虎汤加减;肝肾亏损证,地黄饮子加减;心肾亏虚证,苓桂术甘汤加减。

外治　疳疮,可选用鹅黄散或珍珠散敷于患处。横痃、杨梅结毒未溃时,选用冲和膏,醋、酒各半调成糊状外敷;溃破时,先用五五丹掺在疮面上,外盖玉红膏;待其腐脓涤尽,再用生肌散掺在疮面,盖红玉膏。杨梅疮,可用土茯苓、蛇床子、川椒、蒲公英、莱菔子、白鲜皮煎汤外洗。

1.9.7　艾滋病

艾滋病全称是获得性免疫缺陷综合征,是由人类免疫缺陷病毒(简称 HIV)所致的传染病。属于中医"疫疠"、"虚劳"、"瘰疬"、"癥瘕"等范围。

【诊断】

临床表现,潜伏期长短不一,可由 6 个月至 5 年或更久。感染 HIV 后,由于细胞免疫缺陷的程度不同,临床症状可分为三个阶段:艾滋病感染期、艾滋病相关综合征期、艾滋病期。

免疫学检查、HIV 检测、HIV 抗体检测可明确诊断。

【治疗】

艾滋病的治疗目前尚无特效的疗法。西医的免疫调节剂、抗病毒制剂及综合疗法的实施已能部分控制病情的发展,延长患者的存活时间,提高患者的生存质量;中医中药和其他自然疗法已运用于艾滋病的预防和治疗,抗 HIV 病毒及提高机体免疫功能的中药得以筛选,并推向临床作为辨证论治基础上辨病用药的有效治疗手段,针灸的整体调节功能在治疗中也能发挥一定的作用。

(1)辨证施治　肺卫受邪证,银翘散或荆防败毒散加减;肺肾阴虚证,百合固金汤合瓜蒌贝母汤加虎杖、夏枯草、土大黄等;脾胃虚弱证,补中益气汤合参苓白术散加土茯苓、田基黄、猫爪草等;脾肾亏虚证,肾气丸合四神丸加猪苓、炙甘草等;气虚血瘀证,补阳还五汤、犀角地黄汤合消瘰丸加减;窍闭痰蒙证,用安宫牛黄丸、紫雪丹、至宝丹。若为寒甚者,用苏合香丸豁痰开窍。痰闭清除后,缓则治其本,可用生脉散益气养阴。

(2)常用有效中药对症治疗

①抗 HIV 有效的中药:甘草、人参、党参、黄芪、白术、茯苓、当归、大枣、枸杞子、杜仲、淫羊藿、苦参、柴胡、刺五加、香菇、丹参、黄连、金银花、黄芩、天花粉、紫花地丁等。

②促进单核细胞吞噬能力的中药:仙灵脾、五加皮、白术、黄精、灵芝、蒲公英、银花、丹参、桃仁、赤芍、川芎、香菇、云苓、甘草等。

③促进巨噬细胞吞噬作用的中药:灵芝、猪苓、香菇、当归、地黄、蝮蛇、仙灵脾、补骨脂、刺五加、杜仲等。

④增加 T 细胞的中药:白术、苡仁、黄精、天冬、女贞子、仙灵脾等。

⑤提高细胞免疫力的中药:阿胶、菟丝子、仙灵脾、旱莲草、当归、红花、仙鹤草、丹参、生地、女贞子、枸杞子、白芍、川芎、五味子、银花、黄连等。

⑥提高体液免疫能力的中药:丹参、红花、川芎、当归、仙

鹤草、生地、女贞子、枸杞子、白芍、银花、五味子等。

⑦延长抗体存活及促进其生成的中药：麦冬、玄参、沙参、鳖甲、鸡血藤、阿胶、女贞子等。

⑧延长抗体存活时间：肉桂、附子、仙茅、仙灵脾、锁阳、菟丝子能促进抗体生成，具提高淋巴细胞转化作用。

第 2 章　骨伤科学

中医骨伤科学是在中医药理论指导下,研究和防治骨、关节及其周围软组织损伤性疾病的一门学科。主要内容包括损伤和骨疾病两部分。损伤主要有骨折、脱位、筋伤、损伤内证等,主要由外力伤害、外感六淫邪毒、内在正气亏虚所造成。骨疾病范围较广,包括骨先天性畸形、骨痈疽、骨与关节结核、骨关节痹证、痿证、筋挛、骨关节退行性疾病、骨软骨病、代谢性骨病、骨肿瘤等疾病。骨疾病多由于先天肾精亏虚,后天肾元失充,骨骼空虚,邪毒入侵所致。

2.1　骨折

骨折是指在外力作用下,骨的连续性或完整性发生破坏,其临床症状主要表现为局部疼痛、肿胀、功能障碍、急性异常活动和骨擦音等。骨折是临床上常见的多发性、损伤性疾病。长期以来,中医治疗骨折形成了系统的理论和丰富的临床诊治经验,在骨折整复手法、夹板固定、功能锻炼和中药治疗方面独具特色,疗效显著。

【病因病机】

直接暴力、间接暴力、肌肉强直拉力和慢性劳损等外力伤害作用于人体,可造成骨折。骨折后多发生移位,骨折移位的方式有五种,即:成角移位、侧方移位、缩短移位、分离移位和旋转移位,临床上常合并存在。

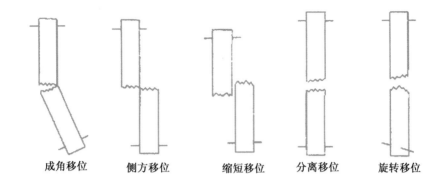

成角移位　　侧方移位　　缩短移位　　分离移位　　旋转移位

图 9　骨折移位的五种方式

骨折的分类:①根据骨折是否与外界相通分为:闭合性骨折和开放性骨折。②根据骨折损伤的程度可分为单纯骨折、复杂骨折、不完全骨折和完全骨折。③根据骨折线的形态分为横断骨折、斜形骨折、螺旋形骨折、粉碎性骨折、嵌插骨折、压缩骨折、裂缝骨折、青枝骨折和骨骺分离。④根据骨折整复后的稳定程度分为:稳定骨折和不稳定骨折。⑤根据骨折发生的时间分为新鲜骨折和陈旧性骨折。⑥根据骨折发生前骨质是否正常分为外伤性骨折和病理性骨折。

骨折的并发症:人体遭受暴力后,除发生骨折外,还可能发生下列全身或局部并发症:①外伤性休克。②感染,开放性骨折易于发生感染。③内脏损伤,可造成肺、肝脾、膀胱、尿道等脏器损伤。④重要动脉损伤。⑤缺血性肌痉挛。⑥脊髓损伤。⑦周围神经损伤。⑧脂肪栓塞。⑨坠积性肺炎。⑩褥疮。⑪尿路感染和结石。⑫损伤性骨化。⑬损伤性关节炎。⑭关节僵硬。⑮缺血性骨坏死。⑯迟发性畸形等。

【诊断】

大多数骨折只引起局部症状,严重骨折和多发性骨折可导致全身反应。

局部表现：

（1）骨折的一般表现　为局部疼痛、肿胀和功能障碍。

（2）骨折的特有体征　①畸形：骨折移位可使患肢外形发生改变，主要表现为缩短、成角或旋转畸形。②异常活动：正常情况下不能活动的部位，骨折后出现不正常的活动。③骨擦音或骨擦感：骨折后，两骨折断端相互摩擦时，可产生骨擦音或骨擦感。

骨折X线检查对骨折的诊断和治疗有重要价值。可以显示临床上难以发现的不完全性骨折、深部骨折、关节内骨折和小的撕脱性骨折等。

【治疗】

骨折的治疗原则包括复位、固定和功能锻炼。

（1）复位　将移位的骨折恢复正常或接近正常的解剖关系，重建骨的支架作用。手法复位：是指医生用指、掌、腕、臂或者身体其他部位的力量结合器械，随证使用各种手法技巧，作用于患者患部及穴位，达到治病疗伤、整骨正位的一种治疗方法。适用于骨折、脱位、筋伤等损伤疾患。正骨基础手法：①拔伸牵引。②旋转。③折顶。④回旋。⑤端提。⑥捺正。⑦分骨。⑧屈伸。⑨纵压。

切开复位：手术切开骨折部位软组织，暴露骨折段，在直视下进行骨折复位。

（2）固定　包括外固定和内固定。外固定有夹板固定、石膏固定和持续牵引三种。

①夹板固定：是利用具有一定弹性的柳木板、竹板或塑料板制成长宽合适的小夹板，在适当的位置加固定垫，绑在骨折部肢体的外面，外扎横带，来固定骨折。夹板固定的指征：适用于四肢

闭合性管状骨骨折,但股骨骨折因大腿肌肉牵引力大,需要结合持续骨牵引;四肢开放性骨折,创口小,经处理创口已基本愈合者;四肢陈旧性骨折,仍适合于手法复位者。夹板固定能够有效地防止骨折发生成角、旋转和侧方移位。由于横带和固定垫的压力可使残余的骨折端侧方或成角移位进一步校正;夹板一般不固定在骨折的上下两个关节,便于及早进行功能锻炼,促进骨折愈合,防止关节僵硬。因而具有固定可靠、骨折愈合快、功能恢复好、并发症少的优点。

②石膏固定:适用于开放性骨折清创缝合后;某些特殊部位如脊柱的骨折;某些骨折切开复位内固定术后;矫形术后以及骨痈疽患肢的固定。

③持续牵引:包括皮肤牵引、布托牵引和骨牵引。

(3)功能锻炼　能够促进全身和局部的气血循环、脏腑功能协调统一;防止废用性肌肉萎缩、骨质疏松、关节强直、瘢痕粘连;在有效的固定力下,利用肌肉的弛张、拮抗、挤压作用使复位的骨折趋于稳定;有助于肢体功能更快地恢复。骨伤科的功能锻炼贯彻局部与整体兼顾、动静结合的治疗原则,是促使功能恢复的一种有效手段。

2.2　脱位

脱位是指构成关节的骨端关节面脱离正常的位置,且发生关节功能障碍,其临床症状有局部疼痛、肿胀、功能障碍、关节畸形、关节盂空虚、弹性固定等。

【病因病机】

脱位的病因主要是外力伤害,慢性劳损等。

脱位的分类：①按照脱位的原因分为外伤性脱位、病理性脱位和习惯性脱位。②按脱位的程度可分为部分性脱位和完全性脱位。③按脱位的方向分为前脱位、后脱位、上脱位、下脱位和中心性脱位。④按脱位后的时间分为新鲜性脱位、陈旧性脱位。⑤按脱位关节是否与外界相通分为闭合性脱位和开放性脱位。

脱位的并发症：骨折、血管损伤、神经损伤、缺血性骨坏死、损伤性骨化和创伤性关节炎。

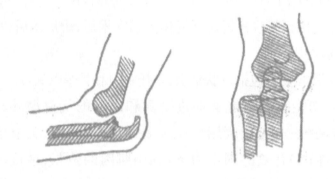

图 10　肘关节后脱位合并桡侧脱位畸形

【诊断】

根据病史，局部肿胀、疼痛、关节畸形、弹性固定、活动障碍，触及关节囊空虚或脱出的关节头一般不难诊断，X 线摄片可明确脱位的方向和类型。

【治疗】

脱位的治疗主要有手法整复、固定、功能锻炼和药物疗法。

手法复位包括拔伸牵引、屈伸、端提等方法，根据脱位的关节不同采用不同的手法。脱位的固定包括布托固定、绷带固定、夹板固定等方法。早期复位后脱位关节可作适度的活动，解除固定后应积极主动锻炼关节功能，但禁止作粗暴动作。药物总以活血化瘀、舒筋活络方法治疗。

2.3 筋 伤

筋伤是指由于扭、挫、刺、割、劳损等原因使皮肤、肌肉、筋膜、肌腱、韧带等软组织,以及软骨、周围神经、较大的血管发生的损伤。

【病因病机】

外来暴力、肌肉强力牵拉、慢性劳损、外感六淫邪毒以及患者素体虚弱均可导致筋伤的发生。

筋伤的分类:①按受伤的性质分为扭伤、挫伤。②按受伤的程度分为撕脱伤、断裂伤、骨错缝。③按受伤的病程分为急性筋伤、慢性筋伤。④按受伤后皮肤黏膜有无破裂分为开放性损伤和闭合性损伤。

筋伤的并发症主要有:撕脱骨折、神经损伤、骨化性肌炎、关节内游离气体和骨性关节炎等。

【诊断】

有劳损病史,局部疼痛,活动障碍,病程长者可有肌肉萎缩,局部感觉障碍等,局部压痛,一般排除骨折、脱位和局部感染。

【治疗】

对于筋伤的治疗可采用理筋手法、针灸疗法、小针刀疗法、牵引疗法、物理疗法以及药物疗法等治疗。

常用的理筋疗法有轻度按摩法、深度按摩法、揉法、拨络法、擦法、滚法、击打法、拿捏法、点穴法、屈伸法、旋转摇晃法、腰部背伸法、按压与踩跷法、抖法、搓法等。

药物以活血化瘀、舒筋活络法治疗。

2.4 损伤内证

损伤内证是指脏腑损伤所引起的气血、脏腑、经络功能紊乱,其主要类型有损伤出血、损伤疼痛、损伤发热、损伤腹胀、损伤昏厥等。

【病因病机】

损伤出血是由于暴力作用于人体,引起经脉破损,血溢脉外。按出血的部位可分为外出血和内出血;按出血量可分为小量、中量、大量出血。伤后血热妄行,亦可引起五官九窍出血。出血较多者可导致血虚证候。

损伤疼痛是指外力伤害人体而引起气血损伤,气机阻滞或瘀血凝聚,不通则痛。一般腰部闪挫多为气滞,各种挫伤多为血瘀,其他损伤多为气滞血瘀并见。伤后正气受损,外邪入侵也可导致疼痛。

损伤发热主要是指受伤积瘀或感受邪毒而生热。

损伤腹胀指外伤后胃肠道内气体积聚,气机阻滞而出现腹部胀满证候。

【诊断】

有明确的外伤史。损伤出血,外出血可见血液自伤口或五官九窍流出,内出血发生在肢体可见肢体肿胀疼痛,发生在胸腹等体腔,则出现胸腹疼痛、面色苍白、体弱无力。

损伤疼痛可表现为胀痛、刺痛、酸痛,郁而化热或感染邪毒则表现为红肿热痛。

损伤发热,瘀血发热多在伤后一日出现,无寒颤,可见血肿。感染邪毒发热多为高热,伴寒颤,可见邪毒感染灶。血虚发热多在午后发热，伴头目眩晕症状。

【治疗】

损伤出血应急救止血、补充血容量、益气固脱。

损伤疼痛根据不同证候应用活血理气、祛风散寒、清热解毒法治疗。

损伤发热，辨证施治，采用活血、解毒、养血疗法治疗。

损伤腹痛，根据不同证候采用攻下逐瘀、理气消滞、补脾益气法治疗。

手术疗法，出血者行血管结扎、修补术，破裂脏器修补术等。

2.5　骨病

骨病范围很广，包括骨先天性畸形、骨痈疽、骨关节退行性疾病、骨软骨病、骨肿瘤等疾病。

【病因病机】

（1）病因　①内因：先天发育情况、年龄、体质、营养状况、脏腑功能状态均可影响骨病的发生。②外因：外感六淫、邪毒感染、慢性劳损、地域因素、毒物与放射线可引起骨损害。

（2）病机　①外邪病机：风邪入侵、寒邪引痛、火邪伤阴导致发病。②气血病机：气滞、血瘀、气虚、血虚均与骨病有关。③经络病机：经络阻隔，气血凝滞，导致骨病发生。④脏腑病机：肾精衰减、肝失疏泄、脾不运化，则筋骨失养，导致骨畸形、骨代谢障碍、关节不利等。

【诊断】

骨病种类很多，临床表现各异。这里仅以骨质疏松为例作一介绍。

骨质疏松多见于老年人,主要临床表现为局限性疼痛、畸形、骨折。疼痛多位于胸段及下腰段椎体。在登高、体位改变时疼痛加重。随着骨质疏松的发展,可发生椎压缩性骨折。出现身高降低,驼背畸形。X 线检查可见到骨密度减低,椎体受压迫出现双凹畸形,或楔形压缩改变,管状骨皮质变薄。氮、双光子矿物质仪可测定骨矿物质含量,可用于早期诊断。

【治疗】

药物治疗　脾气虚弱者,以参苓白术散加减;肾阴不足者,以左归丸加减;肾阳不足,以右归丸加减;气机阻滞,以理气止痛汤加减。中成药以独活寄生丸、健步虎潜丸、六味地黄丸治疗。

外治　外敷伤科消炎膏、正骨水治疗。

其他疗法　西药选用钙剂、性激素、维生素 D、氟化物治疗;还可应用物理疗法。

另外还要加强功能锻炼,注意饮食营养。